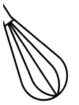

ULCER DIET
COOKBOOK
FOR BEGINNERS

Simple, Nourishing Recipes to Support Your Gut
and manage Symptoms.

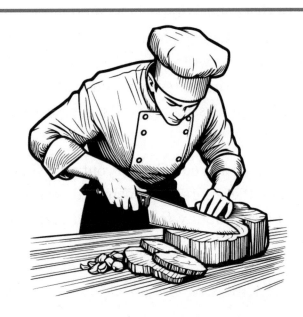

DR ELENA RICHARD

TABLE OF CONTENTS

MAIN DISHES

Introduction

It all started with my younger sister, Mary. I remember the day she called me, her voice tinged with frustration and pain. For weeks, she had been struggling with severe stomach pain, nausea, and constant discomfort. After several visits to the doctor, she was finally diagnosed with a peptic ulcer. The news hit her hard, but it hit me just as hard because I knew the journey ahead wouldn't be easy.

Mary's experience with ulcers was more than just an uncomfortable inconvenience; it affected every part of her life. Meals became a source of anxiety, and she often found herself avoiding food altogether, fearing the flare-ups that would follow. I watched her struggle to find foods that wouldn't irritate her stomach, only to end up with bland, unsatisfying meals that left her feeling deprived.

As someone who has always been passionate about health and nutrition, I couldn't stand by and watch my sister suffer. I dove into research, learning everything I could about ulcers, their causes, and most importantly, how diet could play a role in both triggering and soothing the condition. It became clear that while there were plenty of foods to avoid, there was also a wealth of delicious, nutritious options that could support her health and well-being.

That's when the idea for this book was born. I wanted to create something that would not only help Mary but also anyone else struggling with ulcers. This book is the result of countless hours spent researching, testing recipes, and working closely with Mary to find meals that were both safe for her stomach and satisfying to her palate. I saw firsthand how the right diet could make a significant difference in her quality of life—how it could transform meals from a source of dread into something she could enjoy again.

In the "Ulcer Diet Cookbook for Beginners," you'll find a collection of recipes that have been carefully crafted to be gentle on the stomach without compromising on flavor. Each recipe is designed to help manage symptoms, promote healing, and make your daily meals something to look forward to. Whether you're new to managing an ulcer or have been dealing with it for years, this book is here to guide you through the process.

Understanding Ulcers

Ulcers are open sores that develop on the inner lining of the stomach, upper small intestine, or esophagus. These sores occur when the protective lining of these organs is damaged, allowing digestive acids to eat away at the underlying tissue.

Gastric vs. Duodenal vs. Esophageal Ulcers: Differences and Similarities

Aspect	Gastric Ulcers	Duodenal Ulcers	Esophageal Ulcers
Location	Inner lining of the stomach	Upper part of the small intestine (duodenum)	Lining of the esophagus
Common Causes	- Helicobacter pylori infection	- Helicobacter pylori infection	- Acid reflux (GERD)
	- Long-term use of NSAIDs	- Excessive stomach acid production	- Medications (e.g., bisphosphonates)
			- Infections (e.g., Candida, herpes)
Pain Pattern	- Pain occurs shortly after eating	- Pain occurs 2-3 hours after eating	- Pain often worsens when swallowing
	- Pain may worsen with food	- Pain may be relieved by eating or antacids	- Pain can radiate to the chest or back
Age Group Affected	- More common in older adults	- Can occur at any age, but often in younger adults	- Can occur in any age group, often with GERD

Acid Production	- Normal or low acid levels	- Increased acid production	- Related to acid reflux from the stomach
Bleeding Risk	- Higher risk of bleeding	- Lower risk of bleeding compared to gastric ulcers	- Can lead to bleeding if severe
Healing Response	- Slower to heal due to the constant presence of acid	- Typically heal faster with treatment	- Healing depends on managing the underlying cause
Symptoms	- Nausea and vomiting more common	- May have symptoms at night due to delayed pain	- Painful swallowing (odynophagia)
	- Weight loss more common	- Weight gain or normal weight	- Regurgitation, heartburn
Complications	- Higher risk of developing stomach cancer	- Lower risk of malignancy	- Strictures, Barrett's esophagus
Dietary Influence	- Symptoms may worsen with spicy or fatty foods	- Symptoms may improve with eating or antacids	- Symptoms worsened by acidic, spicy, or hot foods
Diagnosis	- Endoscopy, biopsy for H. pylori, and imaging tests	- Endoscopy, biopsy for H. pylori, and imaging tests	- Endoscopy, barium swallow, pH monitoring
Treatment	- PPIs, H2 blockers, antibiotics (if H. pylori present)	- PPIs, H2 blockers, antibiotics (if H. pylori present)	- PPIs, H2 blockers, antacids, treating underlying cause
Lifestyle Changes	- Avoiding NSAIDs, reducing stress, dietary adjustments	- Avoiding NSAIDs, reducing stress, dietary adjustments	- Elevating the head during sleep, avoiding trigger foods

Summary of Differences:

- **Gastric ulcers** cause pain soon after eating, **duodenal ulcers** typically cause pain hours after eating, and **esophageal ulcers** often cause pain when swallowing.

- **Esophageal ulcers** are strongly linked to acid reflux (GERD) and may lead to complications like strictures or Barrett's esophagus if untreated.

- **Gastric ulcers** have a higher risk of leading to complications like stomach cancer, while **duodenal ulcers** generally have a lower malignancy risk.

Causes and Risk Factors: What You Need to Know

Common Causes of Ulcers

1. **Helicobacter pylori (H. pylori) Infection**

   - **Overview**: H. pylori is a type of bacteria that can live in the digestive tract. Over time, it can cause sores or ulcers in the lining of the stomach or the upper part of the small intestine.

   - **Impact**: H. pylori weaken the protective mucous lining of the stomach, making the tissue more susceptible to damage from stomach acid.

2. **Long-Term Use of Nonsteroidal Anti-Inflammatory Drugs (NSAIDs)**

   - **Overview**: NSAIDs, such as aspirin, ibuprofen, and naproxen, are commonly used to relieve pain and reduce inflammation.

   - **Impact**: These drugs can irritate the stomach lining and interfere with the production of protective mucus, leading to ulcers. Long-term or high-dose use increases the risk.

3. **Excessive Stomach Acid Production**

   - **Overview**: Conditions that lead to increased acid production, such as Zollinger-Ellison syndrome, can result in the formation of ulcers.

   - **Impact**: High levels of stomach acid can erode the lining of the stomach, duodenum, or esophagus, causing ulcers.

4. **Acid Reflux (GERD)**

   - **Overview**: Gastroesophageal reflux disease (GERD) occurs when stomach acid frequently flows back into the esophagus.

- **Impact**: Chronic acid reflux can damage the esophageal lining, leading to the formation of esophageal ulcers.

5. **Infections**

- **Overview**: Certain infections, such as those caused by viruses (e.g., herpes) or fungi (e.g., Candida), can lead to ulceration, especially in the esophagus.

- **Impact**: These infections can weaken the protective barriers in the digestive tract, making it more vulnerable to ulceration.

Risk Factors for Developing Ulcers

1. **Smoking**

- **Impact**: Smoking increases stomach acid production and reduces the production of bicarbonate, which neutralizes acid. It also interferes with blood flow to the stomach lining, impairing healing and increasing the risk of ulcers.

2. **Alcohol Consumption**

- **Impact**: Excessive alcohol intake can irritate and erode the mucous lining of the stomach, leading to inflammation and increased acid production, both of which contribute to ulcer formation.

3. **Stress**

- **Impact**: While stress alone does not cause ulcers, it can exacerbate symptoms and slow down the healing process. Stress may also lead to behaviors, such as smoking or excessive alcohol use, that increase ulcer risk.

4. **Dietary Factors**

- **Impact**: Certain foods and beverages, such as spicy foods, acidic foods, caffeine, and alcohol, can irritate the stomach lining and contribute to the development of ulcers, particularly in individuals with an existing predisposition.

5. **Family History**

- **Impact**: A family history of ulcers may increase your risk, possibly due to shared genetic factors that affect stomach acid production or protective mechanisms in the stomach lining.

6. **Age**

- **Impact**: The risk of developing ulcers increases with age, particularly in individuals over 50. This is partly due to the higher likelihood of H. pylori infection and the increased use of NSAIDs in older adults.

7. **Chronic Conditions**

  - **Impact**: Conditions like chronic obstructive pulmonary disease (COPD), liver disease, and kidney disease can increase the risk of ulcers, either directly or through the medications used to manage these conditions.

Key Takeaways

- **Multi-Factorial Nature**: Ulcers are typically the result of multiple factors working together, such as H. pylori infection combined with NSAID use or smoking.

- **Modifiable Risks**: Many risk factors, such as smoking, alcohol use, and dietary choices, are within your control. Making positive lifestyle changes can significantly reduce your risk of developing ulcers.

- **Importance of Management**: If you have risk factors for ulcers, managing them proactively can prevent the development or worsening of ulcers. This includes regular medical check-ups, appropriate use of medications, and adopting a stomach-friendly diet.

Recognizing Symptoms and Getting Diagnosed

Common Symptoms of Ulcers

1. **Burning or Gnawing Pain**

  - **Location**: This pain is usually felt in the upper abdomen, between the chest and belly button.

  - **Timing**: The pain may occur when the stomach is empty, such as between meals or during the night. It can last from a few minutes to several hours.

  - **Relief**: The pain might be temporarily relieved by eating, drinking milk, or taking antacids, but it often returns.

2. **Bloating and Fullness**

  - **Feeling of Fullness**: Many people with ulcers experience a sensation of being full, even after eating a small amount of food.

- **Bloating**: There may be visible or physical bloating in the stomach area.

3. **Nausea and Vomiting**

   - **Nausea**: Ulcers can cause a persistent feeling of nausea, particularly before or after meals.

   - **Vomiting**: In some cases, vomiting may occur, which could be a sign of a more severe ulcer or a complication.

4. **Loss of Appetite**

   - **Reduced Interest in Food**: Due to the discomfort associated with eating, individuals with ulcers may develop a reduced appetite.

   - **Unintended Weight Loss**: The combination of pain, nausea, and loss of appetite can lead to weight loss.

5. **Heartburn or Acid Reflux**

   - **Burning Sensation**: Some individuals experience heartburn or acid reflux, where stomach acid rises into the esophagus, causing a burning sensation.

   - **Associated Symptoms**: This can be accompanied by a sour taste in the mouth or a feeling of acid backing up into the throat.

6. **Dark or Tarry Stools**

   - **Indication of Bleeding**: Dark, tarry stools (melena) are a sign of bleeding in the upper digestive tract, often due to an ulcer.

   - **Emergency Sign**: This symptom requires immediate medical attention, as it can indicate a serious complication.

7. **Fatigue and Weakness**

   - **Result of Blood Loss**: Chronic bleeding from an ulcer can lead to anemia, causing fatigue, weakness, and pallor.

8. **Vomiting Blood**

   - **Hematemesis**: Vomiting blood, which may appear bright red or resemble coffee grounds, is a sign of a bleeding ulcer and requires urgent medical attention.

When to See a Doctor

- **Persistent Symptoms**: If you experience any of the above symptoms for more than a few days, especially burning pain in the abdomen, it's important to consult a healthcare provider.

- **Severe or Alarming Symptoms**: Immediate medical attention is required if you experience severe abdominal pain, vomiting blood, or notice dark, tarry stools.

Diagnostic Process

1. **Medical History and Physical Examination**

- **Symptom Discussion**: Your doctor will ask about your symptoms, their duration, and any factors that relieve or worsen them.

- **Medication and Lifestyle Review**: They will inquire about your use of NSAIDs, smoking habits, alcohol consumption, and family history of ulcers.

- **Physical Exam**: The doctor may press on your abdomen to check for tenderness or pain.

2. **Diagnostic Tests**

- **Endoscopy (Esophagogastroduodenoscopy - EGD):**

  - **Procedure**: This is the most definitive test for diagnosing ulcers. During an endoscopy, a thin, flexible tube with a camera (endoscope) is inserted through your mouth to examine your stomach, duodenum, and esophagus.

  - **Biopsy**: If an ulcer is found, the doctor may take a small tissue sample (biopsy) to check for H. pylori infection or to rule out cancer.

- **Upper GI Series (Barium Swallow):**

  - **Procedure**: This X-ray test involves drinking a barium solution that coats the lining of your digestive tract, making ulcers visible on the X-ray.

  - **Usage**: It's less commonly used than endoscopy but can be helpful in certain cases.

- **H. pylori Testing:**

  - **Breath Test**: You may be asked to drink a special solution and then breathe into a bag. The breath is analyzed for carbon dioxide produced by H. pylori.

- **Stool Antigen Test**: A sample of your stool can be tested for the presence of H. pylori antigens.

- **Blood Test**: Although less accurate than other tests, a blood test can detect antibodies to H. pylori.

- **Laboratory Tests**:

  - **Complete Blood Count (CBC)**: This test can check for anemia caused by chronic bleeding from an ulcer.

  - **Fecal Occult Blood Test**: This test checks for hidden blood in your stool, which may indicate bleeding from an ulcer.

3. **Differential Diagnosis**

- **Ruling Out Other Conditions**: The doctor may also consider other conditions that could cause similar symptoms, such as gastritis, GERD, or gallbladder disease.

How Certain Foods Affect Ulcers

Foods That May Aggravate Ulcers

1. **Spicy Foods**

- **Effect**: Spices like chili peppers, black pepper, and hot sauces can irritate the stomach lining and increase acid production, which may worsen ulcer pain and discomfort.

- **Recommendation**: It's best to avoid or limit spicy foods, especially during flare-ups.

2. **Caffeinated Beverages**

- **Effect**: Coffee, tea, and caffeinated sodas can stimulate acid production in the stomach, potentially exacerbating ulcer symptoms like pain and heartburn.

- **Recommendation**: Opt for decaffeinated versions or herbal teas that are gentler on the stomach.

3. **Alcohol**

- **Effect**: Alcohol can erode the protective lining of the stomach and increase acid production, leading to irritation and inflammation. It also impairs the healing of existing ulcers.

- **Recommendation**: Limit or avoid alcohol consumption to reduce irritation and promote healing.

4. **Acidic Foods**

   - **Effect**: Foods high in acid, such as citrus fruits (oranges, lemons), tomatoes, and vinegar-based dressings, can irritate the stomach lining and exacerbate symptoms.

   - **Recommendation**: Avoid highly acidic foods and opt for low-acid fruits like bananas, melons, and apples (with the skin removed).

5. **Fatty and Fried Foods**

   - **Effect**: High-fat foods can slow down stomach emptying and increase acid production, leading to discomfort and bloating. Fried foods are particularly hard on the stomach and may trigger symptoms.

   - **Recommendation**: Choose lean proteins and cooking methods like baking, steaming, or grilling instead of frying.

6. **Carbonated Beverages**

   - **Effect**: The carbonation in sodas and sparkling water can cause bloating and increase stomach pressure, which may push acid into the esophagus and aggravate ulcers.

   - **Recommendation**: Stick to still water, herbal teas, or non-carbonated drinks to avoid discomfort.

7. **Chocolate**

   - **Effect**: Chocolate contains both caffeine and a compound called theobromine, both of which can stimulate acid production and relax the lower esophageal sphincter, leading to acid reflux and ulcer irritation.

   - **Recommendation**: Reduce or avoid chocolate, especially during active ulcer flare-ups.

Foods That May Soothe Ulcers

1. **High-Fiber Foods**

   - **Effect**: Fiber can help regulate digestion and prevent the buildup of stomach acid. Whole grains, fruits, and vegetables are excellent sources of fiber that can contribute to overall digestive health.

- **Examples**: Oatmeal, brown rice, whole wheat bread, apples (peeled), and pears.

- **Recommendation**: Incorporate high-fiber foods into your diet gradually to avoid any sudden digestive changes.

2. **Low-Acid Fruits**

- **Effect**: Fruits with low acidity are less likely to irritate the stomach lining. These fruits can also provide essential vitamins and minerals that support healing.

- **Examples**: Bananas, melons, apples (without the skin), and pears.

- **Recommendation**: Include low-acid fruits in your diet as snacks or part of your meals.

3. **Lean Proteins**

- **Effect**: Lean sources of protein are easier on the stomach and can aid in healing by providing the necessary building blocks for tissue repair without increasing acid production.

- **Examples**: Chicken breast, turkey, fish, tofu, and eggs.

- **Recommendation**: Prepare these proteins using gentle cooking methods like baking, steaming, or poaching.

4. **Non-Citrus Vegetables**

- **Effect**: Vegetables that are low in acidity and fiber can help soothe the digestive tract without causing irritation. They are also rich in nutrients that support overall health.

- **Examples**: Broccoli, carrots, green beans, zucchini, and spinach.

- **Recommendation**: Cook vegetables until they are soft to make them easier to digest.

5. **Probiotic-Rich Foods**

- **Effect**: Probiotics are beneficial bacteria that can help balance the gut microbiome, potentially reducing inflammation and promoting healing in the stomach lining.

- **Examples**: Yogurt with live cultures, kefir, sauerkraut, and miso.

- **Recommendation**: Choose low-fat, non-acidic options, and introduce them slowly to your diet.

6. **Herbal Teas**

   - **Effect**: Herbal teas like chamomile, ginger, and licorice root have soothing properties that can reduce inflammation and help manage ulcer symptoms.

   - **Recommendation**: Drink herbal teas warm (not hot) to avoid irritating the stomach lining.

7. **Oatmeal and Porridges**

   - **Effect**: Oatmeal is a bland, high-fiber food that is gentle on the stomach. It can help absorb stomach acid and provide sustained energy without irritating the ulcer.

   - **Recommendation**: Prepare oatmeal with water or low-fat milk and avoid adding acidic toppings like citrus fruits.

8. **Almond Milk**

   - **Effect**: Almond milk is low in acidity and fat, making it a soothing alternative to cow's milk, especially for those who are lactose intolerant or sensitive to dairy.

   - **Recommendation**: Use almond milk in place of regular milk in your cereal, smoothies, or cooking.

Getting Started with an Ulcer-Friendly Diet

Preparing Your Kitchen

Stocking Up on Ulcer-Safe Ingredients

Pantry Staples

- **Whole Grains**

    - Oatmeal

    - Brown rice

    - Quinoa

    - Whole wheat pasta

    - Barley

- **Low-Acid Canned or Packaged Goods**

    - Low-sodium vegetable broth

    - Unsweetened applesauce

    - Canned pears (in juice, not syrup)

    - Canned pumpkin

- **Healthy Oils and Fats**

    - Olive oil

    - Avocado oil

    - Flaxseed oil

- **Herbs and Spices**

    - Ginger

- Turmeric

- Cinnamon

- Dill

- Basil

- Parsley

- **Low-Sodium, Low-Fat Crackers and Breads**

  - Whole wheat crackers

  - Low-sodium rice cakes

  - Whole grain bread

Fresh Produce

- **Low-Acid Fruits**

  - Bananas

  - Melons (e.g., cantaloupe, honeydew)

  - Apples (peeled)

  - Pears

- **Non-Citrus Vegetables**

  - Broccoli

  - Carrots

  - Green beans

  - Zucchini

  - Spinach

  - Sweet potatoes

  - Squash (e.g., butternut, acorn)

- **Herbs and Greens**

  - Lettuce (e.g., romaine, butter lettuce)

- Kale

- Swiss chard

- Fresh parsley and basil

Dairy and Alternatives

- **Low-Fat Dairy**

  - Plain yogurt (with live cultures)

  - Low-fat milk

  - Cottage cheese

  - Low-fat cheese (in moderation)

- **Dairy Alternatives**

  - Almond milk (unsweetened)

  - Oat milk

  - Lactose-free milk

Proteins

- **Lean Meats**

  - Chicken breast (skinless)

  - Turkey breast

  - Lean cuts of beef (e.g., sirloin)

- **Fish**

  - Salmon

  - Cod

  - Tilapia

- **Plant-Based Proteins**

  - Tofu

  - Lentils

- Chickpeas
- Eggs

Beverages

- **Herbal Teas**
  - Chamomile tea
  - Ginger tea
  - Licorice root tea
- **Non-Caffeinated Drinks**
  - Still water
  - Aloe vera juice (diluted, unsweetened)
  - Coconut water

Miscellaneous

- **Probiotic-Rich Foods**
  - Kefir (low-fat)
  - Sauerkraut (low-sodium)
  - Miso (low-sodium)
- **Nut Butters**
  - Almond butter (unsweetened)
  - Peanut butter (natural, unsweetened)

Decoding Food Labels

Understanding Nutritional Information

1. **Serving Size**

   - **What It Is**: The serving size indicates the amount of food that the nutritional information is based on. It is usually listed in common household measurements (e.g., cups, tablespoons) and by weight (e.g., grams, ounces).

   - **Why It Matters**: Understanding serving size helps you gauge how much of the nutrients listed you're actually consuming. If you eat more or less than the serving size, you'll need to adjust the nutritional values accordingly.

2. **Calories**

   - **What It Is**: Calories measure the amount of energy you get from a serving of food.

   - **Why It Matters**: Keeping track of calorie intake is important, especially if you need to manage your weight. Foods high in calories but low in nutrients should be consumed in moderation.

3. **Total Fat**

   - **What It Is**: This section lists the total fat content per serving, including different types of fat like saturated fat and trans fat.

   - **Why It Matters**: Saturated and trans fats can irritate the stomach lining and slow digestion, potentially worsening ulcer symptoms. Opt for foods low in unhealthy fats and higher in healthy fats (like those from olive oil and avocados).

4. **Cholesterol**

   - **What It Is**: Cholesterol is a type of fat found in animal products, and its amount is listed per serving.

   - **Why It Matters**: While dietary cholesterol doesn't directly cause ulcers, a diet high in cholesterol can contribute to other health issues. Choose foods with lower cholesterol levels, especially if you have other risk factors for heart disease.

5. **Sodium**

   - **What It Is**: Sodium, often listed as salt, is a mineral that helps control fluid balance in your body.

- **Why It Matters**: High sodium intake can irritate the stomach lining and worsen ulcer symptoms. It's best to choose low-sodium options (140 mg or less per serving) to reduce irritation.

6. **Total Carbohydrate**

   - **What It Is**: This section lists the total carbohydrates per serving, including dietary fiber and sugars.

   - **Why It Matters**: Carbohydrates provide energy, but it's important to focus on complex carbs that are high in fiber, such as whole grains, to promote smooth digestion. Limit foods high in added sugars, as they can cause rapid blood sugar spikes.

7. **Dietary Fiber**

   - **What It Is**: Fiber is a type of carbohydrate that aids digestion and is not broken down by the body.

   - **Why It Matters**: Fiber helps regulate digestion and can be particularly beneficial for people with ulcers by reducing stomach acid levels. Look for foods high in fiber, aiming for at least 3 grams of fiber per serving.

8. **Sugars**

   - **What It Is**: This includes both naturally occurring sugars (found in fruits and dairy) and added sugars (sugars added during processing).

   - **Why It Matters**: High intake of added sugars can contribute to weight gain and digestive discomfort. Choose foods with low added sugar content, ideally 5 grams or less per serving.

9. **Protein**

   - **What It Is**: Protein is a macronutrient essential for building and repairing tissues.

   - **Why It Matters**: Protein is important for healing, especially in the context of ulcers. Opt for lean protein sources that are easy on the stomach, such as chicken, fish, tofu, and legumes.

10. **Vitamins and Minerals**

- **What It Is**: This section includes essential vitamins and minerals like Vitamin D, calcium, iron, and potassium.

- **Why It Matters**: These nutrients are important for overall health. For ulcer management, focus on foods rich in calcium (which can help reduce stomach acid) and iron (important if you have anemia from ulcer-related blood loss).

Additional Tips for Reading Nutrition Labels

- **Ingredients List**: The ingredients are listed in order of quantity, from highest to lowest. Look for simple, whole-food ingredients and avoid products with long lists of unfamiliar or processed ingredients.

- **"Low," "Free," "Reduced" Claims**: Be cautious of claims like "low-fat," "fat-free," or "reduced sodium." These products may still contain other ingredients that could irritate your stomach, such as added sugars or artificial additives.

- **Daily Value (%DV)**: The %DV tells you how much of a nutrient in a serving of food contributes to a daily diet. For example, 5% DV or less is considered low, and 20% DV or more is considered high. Use this as a guide to gauge whether a food is high or low in a particular nutrient.

- **Avoid Hidden Sources of Irritants**: Be aware of hidden sources of caffeine, alcohol, and acidic ingredients like citric acid or vinegar, which can be present in packaged foods and may exacerbate ulcer symptoms.

60-Day Meal Plan

Day	Breakfast	Lunch	Dinner	Snack/Light Bite
1	Creamy Oatmeal with Banana	Mashed Potato Soup	Baked Chicken Breast with Herbs	Baked Eggplant Slices
2	Poached Egg on Toast	Carrot and Ginger Soup	Grilled Salmon with Dill	Baked Acorn Squash
3	Boiled Egg and Avocado Toast	Cream of Broccoli Soup	Steamed White Fish with Lemon	Baked Zucchini Boats
4	Plain Yogurt with Honey	Cream of Celery Soup	Chicken and Rice Casserole	Baked Parsnip Chips
5	Scrambled Eggs with Cheese	Vegetable Broth with Rice	Baked Tofu Squares	Baked Plantain Slices
6	Banana Smoothie	Cream of Asparagus Soup	Baked Cod with Herbs	Baked Sweet Potato Fries
7	Vegetable Frittata	Cream of Carrot Soup	Grilled Chicken Skewers	Baked Lotus Root Chips
8	Poached Eggs Florentine	Cream of Cauliflower Soup	Grilled Halibut	Baked Taro Chips

9	Baked Apple with Cinnamon	Cream of Potato Leek Soup	Poached Chicken Breast	Baked Yam Wedges
10	Gluten-Free Pancakes (Custom)	Vegetable and Noodle Soup	Baked Tilapia Fillet	Baked Delicata Squash Rings
11	Dairy-Free Smoothie (Custom)	Butternut Squash Soup	Spinach and Cheese Quiche	Baked Sunchoke Chips
12	Quick Scrambled Eggs (Custom)	Cream of Zucchini Soup	Baked Salmon Fillet	Baked Kohlrabi Fries
13	Creamy Oatmeal with Banana	Vegetable and Chickpea Stew	Grilled Tofu Steaks	Baked Turnip Fries
14	Poached Egg on Toast	Cream of Tomato Soup (no seeds)	Baked Chicken Thighs	Baked Carrot Chips
15	Boiled Egg and Avocado Toast	Cream of Spinach Soup	Steamed Mussels in White Wine	Grilled Eggplant Rounds
16	Plain Yogurt with Honey	Vegetable and White Bean Soup	Baked Cod with Breadcrumbs	Steamed Watercress
17	Scrambled Eggs with Cheese	Vegetable and Orzo Soup	Steamed Baby Potatoes	Grilled Polenta Squares
18	Banana Smoothie	Cream of Fennel Soup	Grilled Salmon with Dill	Steamed Fiddlehead Ferns

19	Vegetable Frittata	Vegetable and Millet Soup	Grilled Chicken Skewers	Steamed Pea Shoots
20	Poached Eggs Florentine	Cream of Parsnip Soup	Baked Tilapia Fillet	Steamed Sea Beans
21	Baked Apple with Cinnamon	Cream of Celeriac Soup	Poached Chicken Breast	Steamed Baby Carrots
22	Gluten-Free Smoothie (Custom)	Vegetable and Quinoa Soup	Baked Salmon Fillet	Grilled Papaya Slices
23	Dairy-Free Pancakes (Custom)	Cream of Artichoke Soup	Baked Cod with Herbs	Grilled Mango Cheeks
24	Quick Scrambled Eggs (Custom)	Vegetable and Farro Soup	Grilled Halibut	Grilled Honeydew Melon Wedges
25	Creamy Oatmeal with Banana	Cream of Kohlrabi Soup	Baked Chicken Thighs	Grilled Starfruit Slices
26	Poached Egg on Toast	Mashed Potato Soup	Steamed Mussels in White Wine	Grilled Guava Halves
27	Boiled Egg and Avocado Toast	Carrot and Ginger Soup	Baked Chicken Breast with Herbs	Grilled Dragon Fruit Slices
28	Plain Yogurt with Honey	Cream of Broccoli Soup	Grilled Salmon with Dill	Grilled Kiwi Halves

29	Scrambled Eggs with Cheese	Cream of Celery Soup	Steamed White Fish with Lemon	Grilled Lychee Halves
30	Banana Smoothie	Vegetable Broth with Rice	Chicken and Rice Casserole	Grilled Persimmon Wedges
31	Vegetable Frittata	Cream of Asparagus Soup	Baked Tofu Squares	Baked Plantain Slices
32	Poached Eggs Florentine	Cream of Carrot Soup	Baked Cod with Herbs	Baked Acorn Squash
33	Baked Apple with Cinnamon	Cream of Cauliflower Soup	Grilled Chicken Skewers	Baked Zucchini Boats
34	Gluten-Free Pancakes (Custom)	Cream of Potato Leek Soup	Poached Chicken Breast	Baked Parsnip Chips
35	Dairy-Free Smoothie (Custom)	Vegetable and Noodle Soup	Grilled Tofu Steaks	Baked Yam Wedges
36	Quick Scrambled Eggs (Custom)	Butternut Squash Soup	Baked Chicken Thighs	Baked Sweet Potato Fries
37	Creamy Oatmeal with Banana	Cream of Zucchini Soup	Baked Salmon Fillet	Baked Lotus Root Chips
38	Poached Egg on Toast	Vegetable and Chickpea Stew	Grilled Halibut	Baked Taro Chips
39	Boiled Egg and Avocado Toast	Cream of Tomato Soup (no seeds)	Steamed Mussels in White Wine	Baked Delicata Squash Rings

40	Plain Yogurt with Honey	Cream of Spinach Soup	Grilled Chicken Skewers	Baked Sunchoke Chips
41	Scrambled Eggs with Cheese	Vegetable and White Bean Soup	Baked Tilapia Fillet	Baked Kohlrabi Fries
42	Banana Smoothie	Vegetable and Orzo Soup	Baked Chicken Breast with Herbs	Baked Turnip Fries
43	Vegetable Frittata	Cream of Fennel Soup	Grilled Salmon with Dill	Baked Carrot Chips
44	Poached Eggs Florentine	Vegetable and Millet Soup	Steamed White Fish with Lemon	Grilled Eggplant Rounds
45	Baked Apple with Cinnamon	Cream of Parsnip Soup	Chicken and Rice Casserole	Steamed Watercress
46	Gluten-Free Smoothie (Custom)	Cream of Celeriac Soup	Baked Tofu Squares	Steamed Fiddlehead Ferns
47	Dairy-Free Pancakes (Custom)	Vegetable and Quinoa Soup	Baked Cod with Herbs	Steamed Sea Beans
48	Quick Scrambled Eggs (Custom)	Cream of Artichoke Soup	Grilled Halibut	Steamed Pea Shoots
49	Creamy Oatmeal with Banana	Vegetable and Farro Soup	Baked Chicken Thighs	Grilled Papaya Slices

50	Poached Egg on Toast	Cream of Kohlrabi Soup	Baked Salmon Fillet	Grilled Mango Cheeks
51	Boiled Egg and Avocado Toast	Mashed Potato Soup	Grilled Chicken Skewers	Grilled Honeydew Melon Wedges
52	Plain Yogurt with Honey	Carrot and Ginger Soup	Poached Chicken Breast	Grilled Starfruit Slices
53	Scrambled Eggs with Cheese	Cream of Broccoli Soup	Baked Tilapia Fillet	Grilled Guava Halves
54	Banana Smoothie	Cream of Celery Soup	Grilled Tofu Steaks	Grilled Dragon Fruit Slices
55	Vegetable Frittata	Vegetable Broth with Rice	Baked Chicken Thighs	Grilled Kiwi Halves
56	Poached Eggs Florentine	Cream of Asparagus Soup	Grilled Salmon with Dill	Grilled Lychee Halves
57	Baked Apple with Cinnamon	Cream of Carrot Soup	Baked Cod with Herbs	Grilled Persimmon Wedges
58	Gluten-Free Pancakes (Custom)	Cream of Cauliflower Soup	Grilled Chicken Skewers	Baked Plantain Slices
59	Dairy-Free Smoothie (Custom)	Cream of Potato Leek Soup	Poached Chicken Breast	Baked Acorn Squash
60	Quick Scrambled Eggs (Custom)	Vegetable and Noodle Soup	Baked Tofu Squares	Baked Zucchini Boats

Breakfast Recipes

Creamy Oatmeal with Banana

Prep Time: 5 minutes | **Cooking Time:** 10 minutes | **Total Time:** 15 minutes | **Serving:** 2 | **Difficulty:** Easy

Ingredients:

- 1 cup rolled oats
- 2 cups water or low-fat milk
- 1 ripe banana, sliced
- 1 tablespoon honey
- 1/2 teaspoon ground cinnamon
- A pinch of salt
- Optional toppings: chopped nuts, raisins, or additional banana slices

Instructions:

1. In a medium saucepan, bring the water or milk to a boil.
2. Stir in the oats, reduce heat to low, and simmer for 5-7 minutes, stirring occasionally, until the oats are soft and creamy.
3. Remove from heat and stir in the banana slices, honey, cinnamon, and salt.
4. Divide the oatmeal into bowls and add optional toppings if desired.
5. Serve immediately.

Nutritional Value:

240 calories | 5g fat | 1g saturated fat | 0mg cholesterol | 10mg sodium | 44g carbohydrate | 6g fiber | 12g sugar | 6g protein | 150mg calcium | 300mg potassium | 130mg phosphorus | 1.5mg iron | 0mcg vitamin D

Poached Egg on Toast

Prep Time: 5 minutes | **Cooking Time:** 10 minutes | **Total Time:** 15 minutes | **Serving:** 1 | **Difficulty:** Easy

Ingredients:

- 1 large egg
- 1 slice whole grain bread
- 1 teaspoon white vinegar
- Salt and pepper, to taste
- Optional: butter or margarine for spreading

Instructions:

1. Fill a saucepan with water and add the vinegar; bring to a simmer over medium heat.

2. Crack the egg into a small bowl. Carefully slide the egg into the simmering water.

3. Poach the egg for 3-4 minutes until the white is set and the yolk remains soft.

4. Meanwhile, toast the bread to your desired level of crispness.

5. Remove the poached egg with a slotted spoon and place it on the toast.

6. Season with salt and pepper. Serve immediately with optional butter or margarine spread on the toast.

Nutritional Value:

170 calories | 7g fat | 2g saturated fat | 186mg cholesterol | 240mg sodium | 17g carbohydrate | 2g fiber | 1g sugar | 8g protein | 50mg calcium | 100mg potassium | 85mg phosphorus | 1mg iron | 1.1mcg vitamin D

Boiled Egg and Avocado Toast

Prep Time: 5 minutes | **Cooking Time:** 10 minutes | **Total Time:** 15 minutes | **Serving:** 1 | **Difficulty:** Easy

Ingredients:

- 1 large egg

- 1/2 ripe avocado, mashed

- 1 slice whole grain bread

- Salt and pepper, to taste

- Optional: lemon juice or red pepper flakes for garnish

Instructions:

1. Place the egg in a saucepan and cover with water. Bring to a boil, then reduce the heat and simmer for 9-12 minutes, depending on your desired level of doneness.

2. While the egg is cooking, toast the bread to your desired level of crispness.

3. Spread the mashed avocado over the toast and season with salt and pepper.

4. Peel the boiled egg, slice it, and arrange the slices on top of the avocado toast.

5. Add optional garnishes like lemon juice or red pepper flakes if desired.

6. Serve immediately.

Nutritional Value:

220 calories | 13g fat | 2g saturated fat | 186mg cholesterol | 220mg sodium | 19g carbohydrate | 5g fiber | 1g sugar | 9g protein | 40mg calcium | 350mg potassium | 110mg phosphorus | 1.5mg iron | 1.1mcg vitamin D

Plain Yogurt with Honey

Prep Time: 2 minutes | **Cooking Time:** 0 minutes | **Total Time:** 2 minutes | **Serving:** 1 | **Difficulty:** Easy

Ingredients:

- 1 cup plain low-fat yogurt
- 1 tablespoon honey
- Optional toppings: fresh fruit, granola, or nuts

Instructions:

1. Spoon the yogurt into a serving bowl.
2. Drizzle the honey over the top.
3. Add any optional toppings if desired.
4. Serve immediately.

Nutritional Value:
150 calories | 2g fat | 1g saturated fat | 10mg cholesterol | 70mg sodium | 28g carbohydrate | 0g fiber | 26g sugar | 6g protein | 200mg calcium | 350mg potassium | 150mg phosphorus | 0.5mg iron | 0mcg vitamin D

Scrambled Eggs with Cheese

Prep Time: 3 minutes | **Cooking Time:** 5 minutes | **Total Time:** 8 minutes | **Serving:** 1 | **Difficulty:** Easy

Ingredients:

- 2 large eggs
- 2 tablespoons low-fat milk
- 1/4 cup shredded low-fat cheese (e.g., cheddar, mozzarella)
- Salt and pepper, to taste
- 1 teaspoon butter or olive oil

Instructions:

1. In a bowl, whisk together the eggs, milk, salt, and pepper.
2. Heat the butter or olive oil in a non-stick skillet over medium heat.
3. Pour the egg mixture into the skillet and cook, stirring frequently, until the eggs are just set.
4. Sprinkle the cheese over the eggs and continue cooking until the cheese melts and the eggs are fully cooked.
5. Serve immediately.

Nutritional Value:
220 calories | 14g fat | 5g saturated fat | 390mg cholesterol | 300mg sodium | 2g carbohydrate | 0g fiber | 1g sugar | 18g protein | 200mg calcium | 250mg potassium | 150mg phosphorus | 2mg iron | 1.4mcg vitamin D

Banana Smoothie

Prep Time: 5 minutes | **Cooking Time:** 0 minutes | **Total Time:** 5 minutes | **Serving:** 1 | **Difficulty:** Easy

Ingredients:

- 1 ripe banana
- 1/2 cup low-fat milk or almond milk
- 1/2 cup plain low-fat yogurt
- 1 tablespoon honey
- 1/4 teaspoon vanilla extract
- Ice cubes (optional)

Instructions:

1. In a blender, combine the banana, milk, yogurt, honey, and vanilla extract.
2. Blend until smooth and creamy.
3. Add ice cubes if you prefer a colder, thicker smoothie.
4. Pour into a glass and serve immediately.

Nutritional Value:

200 calories | 4g fat | 2g saturated fat | 10mg cholesterol | 60mg sodium | 40g carbohydrate | 2g fiber | 28g sugar | 6g protein | 150mg calcium | 400mg potassium | 100mg phosphorus | 1mg iron | 0mcg vitamin D

Vegetable Frittata

Prep Time: 10 minutes | **Cooking Time:** 20 minutes | **Total Time:** 30 minutes | **Serving:** 4 | **Difficulty:** Easy

Ingredients:

- 6 large eggs
- 1/4 cup low-fat milk
- 1/2 cup diced bell peppers
- 1/2 cup chopped spinach
- 1/4 cup diced onions
- 1/4 cup shredded low-fat cheese
- 1 tablespoon olive oil
- Salt and pepper, to taste

Instructions:

1. Preheat your oven to 350°F (175°C).
2. In a large bowl, whisk together the eggs, milk, salt, and pepper.
3. Heat the olive oil in an oven-safe skillet over medium heat. Add the onions and bell peppers, cooking until softened.
4. Stir in the spinach and cook until wilted.
5. Pour the egg mixture over the vegetables in the skillet. Sprinkle with cheese.
6. Transfer the skillet to the preheated oven and bake for 15-20 minutes,

until the frittata is set and slightly golden.

7. Remove from the oven, let cool slightly, then slice and serve.

Nutritional Value:

180 calories | 10g fat | 3g saturated fat | 280mg cholesterol | 220mg sodium | 5g carbohydrate | 1g fiber | 3g sugar | 15g protein | 150mg calcium | 300mg potassium | 120mg phosphorus | 2mg iron | 1.2mcg vitamin D

Poached Eggs Florentine

Prep Time: 5 minutes | **Cooking Time:** 10 minutes | **Total Time:** 15 minutes | **Serving:** 2 | **Difficulty:** Medium

Ingredients:

- 2 large eggs
- 2 cups fresh spinach leaves
- 1 teaspoon white vinegar
- 2 slices whole grain bread
- 1 tablespoon butter
- Salt and pepper, to taste
- Optional: Hollandaise sauce for topping

Instructions:

1. Fill a saucepan with water and add the vinegar; bring to a simmer over medium heat.

2. Crack each egg into a small bowl. Carefully slide the eggs into the simmering water and poach for 3-4 minutes until the whites are set.

3. While the eggs are poaching, toast the bread and sauté the spinach in butter until wilted.

4. Place the sautéed spinach on the toasted bread slices.

5. Remove the poached eggs with a slotted spoon and place them on top of the spinach.

6. Season with salt and pepper, and top with Hollandaise sauce if desired.

7. Serve immediately.

Nutritional Value:

220 calories | 13g fat | 6g saturated fat | 400mg cholesterol | 340mg sodium | 15g carbohydrate | 2g fiber | 2g sugar | 12g protein | 120mg calcium | 250mg potassium | 140mg phosphorus | 1.5mg iron | 1.4mcg vitamin D

Baked Apple with Cinnamon

Prep Time: 5 minutes | **Cooking Time:** 30 minutes | **Total Time:** 35 minutes | **Serving:** 2 | **Difficulty:** Easy

Ingredients:

- 2 medium apples, cored
- 2 tablespoons honey
- 1/2 teaspoon ground cinnamon
- 1/4 teaspoon nutmeg (optional)
- 1 tablespoon unsalted butter, cut into small pieces
- Optional: Chopped nuts or raisins for topping

Instructions:

1. Preheat your oven to 350°F (175°C).
2. Place the cored apples in a baking dish.
3. Drizzle honey into the center of each apple and sprinkle with cinnamon and nutmeg.
4. Place a few small pieces of butter on top of each apple.
5. Bake in the preheated oven for 25-30 minutes, until the apples are tender.
6. Remove from the oven and let cool slightly.
7. Serve warm, topped with optional nuts or raisins if desired.

Nutritional Value:

180 calories | 5g fat | 3g saturated fat | 15mg cholesterol | 20mg sodium | 35g carbohydrate | 5g fiber | 28g sugar | 1g protein | 50mg calcium | 200mg potassium | 20mg phosphorus | 0.3mg iron | 0mcg vitamin D

Soups and Broths

Mashed Potato Soup

Prep Time: 15 minutes | **Cooking Time:** 25 minutes | **Total Time:** 40 minutes | **Serving:** 4 | **Difficulty:** Easy

Ingredients:

- 4 large potatoes, peeled and diced
- 1 medium onion, chopped
- 2 cloves garlic, minced
- 4 cups low-sodium vegetable broth
- 1 cup low-fat milk
- 2 tablespoons unsalted butter
- Salt and pepper, to taste
- Fresh chives, chopped (optional)

Instructions:

1. In a large pot, melt the butter over medium heat. Add the onion and garlic, sautéing until softened, about 5 minutes.

2. Add the diced potatoes and vegetable broth to the pot. Bring to a boil, then reduce the heat and simmer for 20 minutes, or until the potatoes are tender.

3. Use an immersion blender to blend the soup until smooth, or transfer to a blender in batches.

4. Stir in the milk and season with salt and pepper.

5. Simmer for an additional 5 minutes, stirring occasionally.

6. Serve hot, garnished with fresh chives if desired.

Nutritional Value:

200 calories | 7g fat | 4g saturated fat | 15mg cholesterol | 240mg sodium | 30g carbohydrate | 3g fiber | 5g sugar | 4g protein | 150mg calcium | 400mg potassium | 90mg phosphorus | 1mg iron | 0mcg vitamin D

Vegetable Broth with Rice

Prep Time: 10 minutes | **Cooking Time:** 30 minutes | **Total Time:** 40 minutes | **Serving:** 4 | **Difficulty:** Easy

Ingredients:

- 1 cup uncooked brown rice
- 4 cups low-sodium vegetable broth
- 1 medium carrot, diced
- 1 celery stalk, diced
- 1 small onion, diced
- 2 cloves garlic, minced

- 1 tablespoon olive oil
- Salt and pepper, to taste

Instructions:

1. In a large pot, heat the olive oil over medium heat. Add the onion, garlic, carrot, and celery, sautéing until softened, about 5 minutes.

2. Add the vegetable broth and bring to a boil.

3. Stir in the brown rice and reduce the heat to low. Simmer, covered, for 25-30 minutes, until the rice is tender.

4. Season with salt and pepper to taste.

5. Serve hot.

Nutritional Value:
180 calories | 5g fat | 1g saturated fat | 0mg cholesterol | 200mg sodium | 30g carbohydrate | 3g fiber | 4g sugar | 4g protein | 40mg calcium | 250mg potassium | 80mg phosphorus | 1mg iron | 0mcg vitamin D

Carrot and Ginger Soup

Prep Time: 10 minutes | **Cooking Time:** 25 minutes | **Total Time:** 35 minutes | **Serving:** 4 | **Difficulty:** Easy

Ingredients:

- 1 lb carrots, peeled and chopped
- 1 medium onion, chopped
- 2 cloves garlic, minced
- 1 tablespoon fresh ginger, minced
- 4 cups low-sodium vegetable broth
- 1 tablespoon olive oil
- 1/2 cup low-fat coconut milk (optional for creaminess)
- Salt and pepper, to taste

Instructions:

1. In a large pot, heat the olive oil over medium heat. Add the onion, garlic, and ginger, sautéing until fragrant, about 3-4 minutes.

2. Add the chopped carrots and vegetable broth. Bring to a boil, then reduce the heat and simmer for 20 minutes, or until the carrots are tender.

3. Use an immersion blender to puree the soup until smooth, or transfer to a blender in batches.

4. Stir in the coconut milk if using, and season with salt and pepper.

5. Simmer for an additional 5 minutes.

6. Serve hot.

Nutritional Value:
150 calories | 5g fat | 2g saturated fat | 0mg cholesterol | 220mg sodium | 24g carbohydrate | 5g fiber | 9g sugar | 2g protein | 50mg calcium | 400mg potassium | 70mg phosphorus | 1mg iron | 0mcg vitamin

D

Butternut Squash Soup

Prep Time: 15 minutes | **Cooking Time:** 30 minutes | **Total Time:** 45 minutes | **Serving:** 4 | **Difficulty:** Easy

Ingredients:

- 1 medium butternut squash, peeled and cubed
- 1 medium onion, chopped
- 2 cloves garlic, minced
- 4 cups low-sodium vegetable broth
- 1 tablespoon olive oil
- 1/2 teaspoon ground cinnamon
- 1/4 teaspoon ground nutmeg (optional)
- Salt and pepper, to taste
- Fresh parsley, chopped (optional for garnish)

Instructions:

1. In a large pot, heat the olive oil over medium heat. Add the onion and garlic, sautéing until softened, about 5 minutes.

2. Add the cubed butternut squash, cinnamon, nutmeg, and vegetable broth. Bring to a boil, then reduce the heat and simmer for 25-30 minutes, or until the squash is tender.

3. Use an immersion blender to puree the soup until smooth, or transfer to a blender in batches.

4. Season with salt and pepper to taste.

5. Serve hot, garnished with fresh parsley if desired.

Nutritional Value:

180 calories | 6g fat | 1g saturated fat | 0mg cholesterol | 220mg sodium | 32g carbohydrate | 5g fiber | 7g sugar | 3g protein | 80mg calcium | 450mg potassium | 90mg phosphorus | 1mg iron | 0mcg vitamin D

Cream of Celery Soup

Prep Time: 10 minutes | **Cooking Time:** 20 minutes | **Total Time:** 30 minutes | **Serving:** 4 | **Difficulty:** Easy

Ingredients:

- 6 celery stalks, chopped
- 1 medium onion, chopped
- 2 cloves garlic, minced
- 2 tablespoons unsalted butter
- 3 cups low-sodium vegetable broth
- 1 cup low-fat milk
- 2 tablespoons all-purpose flour
- Salt and pepper, to taste

- Fresh parsley, chopped (optional for garnish)

Instructions:

1. In a large pot, melt the butter over medium heat. Add the onion, garlic, and celery, sautéing until softened, about 8 minutes.

2. Sprinkle the flour over the vegetables and stir to coat evenly.

3. Gradually add the vegetable broth, stirring constantly to avoid lumps. Bring to a simmer and cook for 10 minutes.

4. Use an immersion blender to puree the soup until smooth, or transfer to a blender in batches.

5. Stir in the milk and season with salt and pepper to taste.

6. Simmer for an additional 5 minutes.

7. Serve hot, garnished with fresh parsley if desired.

Nutritional Value:
190 calories | 8g fat | 4g saturated fat | 15mg cholesterol | 220mg sodium | 24g carbohydrate | 3g fiber | 6g sugar | 5g protein | 120mg calcium | 350mg potassium | 80mg phosphorus | 1mg iron | 0mcg vitamin D

Cream of Mushroom Soup

Prep Time: 10 minutes | **Cooking Time:** 25 minutes | **Total Time:** 35 minutes | **Serving:** 4 | **Difficulty:** Easy

Ingredients:

- 8 oz mushrooms, sliced
- 1 medium onion, chopped
- 2 cloves garlic, minced
- 2 tablespoons unsalted butter
- 3 cups low-sodium vegetable broth
- 1 cup low-fat milk
- 2 tablespoons all-purpose flour
- Salt and pepper, to taste
- Fresh thyme or parsley, chopped (optional for garnish)

Instructions:

1. In a large pot, melt the butter over medium heat. Add the onion, garlic, and mushrooms, sautéing until the mushrooms release their moisture and are golden brown, about 8 minutes.

2. Sprinkle the flour over the vegetables and stir to coat evenly.

3. Gradually add the vegetable broth, stirring constantly to avoid lumps. Bring to a simmer and cook for 10 minutes.

4. Use an immersion blender to puree the soup until smooth, or transfer to a blender in batches.

5. Stir in the milk and season with salt and pepper to taste.

6. Simmer for an additional 5 minutes.

7. Serve hot, garnished with fresh thyme or parsley if desired.

Nutritional Value:

170 calories | 8g fat | 4g saturated fat | 15mg cholesterol | 230mg sodium | 20g carbohydrate | 3g fiber | 4g sugar | 6g protein | 120mg calcium | 400mg potassium | 90mg phosphorus | 1mg iron | 0mcg vitamin D

Cream of Asparagus Soup

Prep Time: 10 minutes | **Cooking Time:** 20 minutes | **Total Time:** 30 minutes | **Serving:** 4 | **Difficulty:** Easy

Ingredients:

- 1 lb asparagus, trimmed and cut into 1-inch pieces

- 1 medium onion, chopped

- 2 cloves garlic, minced

- 2 tablespoons unsalted butter

- 3 cups low-sodium vegetable broth

- 1 cup low-fat milk

- 2 tablespoons all-purpose flour

- Salt and pepper, to taste

- Fresh dill or chives, chopped (optional for garnish)

Instructions:

1. In a large pot, melt the butter over medium heat. Add the onion, garlic, and asparagus, sautéing until the onion is softened, about 5 minutes.

2. Sprinkle the flour over the vegetables and stir to coat evenly.

3. Gradually add the vegetable broth, stirring constantly to avoid lumps. Bring to a simmer and cook for 10 minutes.

4. Use an immersion blender to puree the soup until smooth, or transfer to a blender in batches.

5. Stir in the milk and season with salt and pepper to taste.

6. Simmer for an additional 5 minutes.

7. Serve hot, garnished with fresh dill or chives if desired.

Nutritional Value:

160 calories | 7g fat | 4g saturated fat | 15mg cholesterol | 220mg sodium | 18g carbohydrate | 3g fiber | 4g sugar | 5g protein | 120mg calcium | 450mg potassium | 80mg phosphorus | 1mg iron | 0mcg vitamin D

Vegetable and Noodle Soup

Prep Time: 10 minutes | **Cooking Time:** 20 minutes | **Total Time:** 30 minutes | **Serving:** 4 | **Difficulty:** Easy

Ingredients:

- 1 cup whole wheat noodles
- 4 cups low-sodium vegetable broth
- 1 medium carrot, diced
- 1 celery stalk, diced
- 1 small zucchini, diced
- 1 small onion, chopped
- 2 cloves garlic, minced
- 1 tablespoon olive oil
- Salt and pepper, to taste
- Fresh parsley, chopped (optional for garnish)

Instructions:

1. In a large pot, heat the olive oil over medium heat. Add the onion, garlic, carrot, and celery, sautéing until softened, about 5 minutes.

2. Add the vegetable broth and bring to a boil.

3. Stir in the noodles and zucchini. Reduce the heat and simmer for 10-12 minutes, or until the noodles are tender.

4. Season with salt and pepper to taste.

5. Serve hot, garnished with fresh parsley if desired.

Nutritional Value:

180 calories | 5g fat | 1g saturated fat | 0mg cholesterol | 240mg sodium | 28g carbohydrate | 4g fiber | 5g sugar | 5g protein | 50mg calcium | 350mg potassium | 80mg phosphorus | 1mg iron | 0mcg vitamin D

Cream of Broccoli Soup

Prep Time: 10 minutes | **Cooking Time:** 20 minutes | **Total Time:** 30 minutes | **Serving:** 4 | **Difficulty:** Easy

Ingredients:

- 1 lb broccoli florets
- 1 medium onion, chopped
- 2 cloves garlic, minced
- 2 tablespoons unsalted butter
- 3 cups low-sodium vegetable broth
- 1 cup low-fat milk
- 2 tablespoons all-purpose flour
- Salt and pepper, to taste
- Fresh parsley, chopped (optional for garnish)

Instructions:

1. In a large pot, melt the butter over medium heat. Add the onion, garlic,

and broccoli, sautéing until the onion is softened, about 5 minutes.

2. Sprinkle the flour over the vegetables and stir to coat evenly.

3. Gradually add the vegetable broth, stirring constantly to avoid lumps. Bring to a simmer and cook for 10 minutes, or until the broccoli is tender.

4. Use an immersion blender to puree the soup until smooth, or transfer to a blender in batches.

5. Stir in the milk and season with salt and pepper to taste.

6. Simmer for an additional 5 minutes.

7. Serve hot, garnished with fresh parsley if desired.

Nutritional Value:

170 calories | 8g fat | 4g saturated fat | 15mg cholesterol | 220mg sodium | 20g carbohydrate | 4g fiber | 6g sugar | 5g protein | 120mg calcium | 400mg potassium | 80mg phosphorus | 1mg iron | 0mcg vitamin D

Cream of Carrot Soup

Prep Time: 10 minutes | **Cooking Time:** 20 minutes | **Total Time:** 30 minutes | **Serving:** 4 | **Difficulty:** Easy

Ingredients:

- 1 lb carrots, peeled and chopped
- 1 medium onion, chopped
- 2 cloves garlic, minced
- 2 tablespoons unsalted butter
- 3 cups low-sodium vegetable broth
- 1 cup low-fat milk
- 2 tablespoons all-purpose flour
- Salt and pepper, to taste
- Fresh parsley, chopped (optional for garnish)

Instructions:

1. In a large pot, melt the butter over medium heat. Add the onion, garlic, and carrots, sautéing until the onion is softened, about 5 minutes.

2. Sprinkle the flour over the vegetables and stir to coat evenly.

3. Gradually add the vegetable broth, stirring constantly to avoid lumps. Bring to a simmer and cook for 10 minutes, or until the carrots are tender.

4. Use an immersion blender to puree the soup until smooth, or transfer to a blender in batches.

5. Stir in the milk and season with salt and pepper to taste.

6. Simmer for an additional 5 minutes.

7. Serve hot, garnished with fresh parsley if desired.

Nutritional Value:

160 calories | 7g fat | 4g saturated fat | 15mg cholesterol | 220mg sodium | 18g carbohydrate | 4g fiber | 6g sugar | 4g protein | 120mg calcium | 400mg potassium | 80mg phosphorus | 1mg iron | 0mcg vitamin D

Cream of Cauliflower Soup

Prep Time: 10 minutes | **Cooking Time:** 20 minutes | **Total Time:** 30 minutes | **Serving:** 4 | **Difficulty:** Easy

Ingredients:

- 1 head cauliflower, chopped into florets
- 1 medium onion, chopped
- 2 cloves garlic, minced
- 2 tablespoons unsalted butter
- 3 cups low-sodium vegetable broth
- 1 cup low-fat milk
- 2 tablespoons all-purpose flour
- Salt and pepper, to taste
- Fresh parsley, chopped (optional for garnish)

Instructions:

1. In a large pot, melt the butter over medium heat. Add the onion, garlic, and cauliflower, sautéing until the onion is softened, about 5 minutes.
2. Sprinkle the flour over the vegetables and stir to coat evenly.
3. Gradually add the vegetable broth, stirring constantly to avoid lumps. Bring to a simmer and cook for 10 minutes, or until the cauliflower is tender.
4. Use an immersion blender to puree the soup until smooth, or transfer to a blender in batches.
5. Stir in the milk and season with salt and pepper to taste.
6. Simmer for an additional 5 minutes.
7. Serve hot, garnished with fresh parsley if desired.

Nutritional Value:

160 calories | 8g fat | 4g saturated fat | 15mg cholesterol | 220mg sodium | 15g carbohydrate | 3g fiber | 5g sugar | 4g protein | 120mg calcium | 300mg potassium | 80mg phosphorus | 1mg iron | 0mcg vitamin D

Cream of Potato Leek Soup

Prep Time: 10 minutes | **Cooking Time:** 30 minutes | **Total Time:** 40 minutes | **Serving:** 4 | **Difficulty:** Easy

Ingredients:

- 4 large potatoes, peeled and diced

- 2 leeks, cleaned and sliced (white and light green parts only)

- 2 cloves garlic, minced

- 2 tablespoons unsalted butter

- 4 cups low-sodium vegetable broth

- 1 cup low-fat milk

- Salt and pepper, to taste

- Fresh chives, chopped (optional for garnish)

Instructions:

1. In a large pot, melt the butter over medium heat. Add the leeks and garlic, sautéing until softened, about 5 minutes.

2. Add the diced potatoes and vegetable broth to the pot. Bring to a boil, then reduce the heat and simmer for 20-25 minutes, or until the potatoes are tender.

3. Use an immersion blender to puree the soup until smooth, or transfer to a blender in batches.

4. Stir in the milk and season with salt and pepper to taste.

5. Simmer for an additional 5 minutes.

6. Serve hot, garnished with fresh chives if desired.

Nutritional Value:
210 calories | 7g fat | 4g saturated fat | 15mg cholesterol | 240mg sodium | 35g carbohydrate | 4g fiber | 5g sugar | 4g protein | 150mg calcium | 400mg potassium | 100mg phosphorus | 1mg iron | 0mcg vitamin D

Vegetable and Lentil Soup

Prep Time: 15 minutes | **Cooking Time:** 30 minutes | **Total Time:** 45 minutes | **Serving:** 4 | **Difficulty:** Easy

Ingredients:

- 1 cup dried lentils, rinsed

- 1 medium carrot, diced

- 1 celery stalk, diced

- 1 small zucchini, diced

- 1 small onion, chopped

- 2 cloves garlic, minced

- 1 tablespoon olive oil

- 4 cups low-sodium vegetable broth

- 1 teaspoon ground cumin

- Salt and pepper, to taste

- Fresh parsley, chopped (optional for garnish)

Instructions:

1. In a large pot, heat the olive oil over medium heat. Add the onion, garlic, carrot, and celery, sautéing until softened, about 5 minutes.

2. Add the lentils, zucchini, vegetable broth, and cumin to the pot. Bring to a boil, then reduce the heat and simmer for 25-30 minutes, or until the lentils are tender.

3. Season with salt and pepper to taste.

4. Serve hot, garnished with fresh parsley if desired.

Nutritional Value:

240 calories | 5g fat | 1g saturated fat | 0mg cholesterol | 220mg sodium | 40g carbohydrate | 8g fiber | 4g sugar | 12g protein | 60mg calcium | 500mg potassium | 150mg phosphorus | 3mg iron | 0mcg vitamin D

Cream of Zucchini Soup

Prep Time: 10 minutes | **Cooking Time:** 20 minutes | **Total Time:** 30 minutes | **Serving:** 4 | **Difficulty:** Easy

Ingredients:

- 4 medium zucchinis, sliced

- 1 medium onion, chopped

- 2 cloves garlic, minced

- 2 tablespoons unsalted butter

- 3 cups low-sodium vegetable broth

- 1 cup low-fat milk

- Salt and pepper, to taste

- Fresh dill, chopped (optional for garnish)

Instructions:

1. In a large pot, melt the butter over medium heat. Add the onion, garlic, and zucchini, sautéing until the onion is softened, about 5 minutes.

2. Add the vegetable broth and bring to a boil. Reduce the heat and simmer for 15 minutes, or until the zucchini is tender.

3. Use an immersion blender to puree the soup until smooth, or transfer to a blender in batches.

4. Stir in the milk and season with salt and pepper to taste.

5. Simmer for an additional 5 minutes.

6. Serve hot, garnished with fresh dill if desired.

Nutritional Value:

150 calories | 7g fat | 4g saturated fat | 15mg cholesterol | 220mg sodium | 15g carbohydrate | 2g fiber | 5g sugar | 4g protein | 120mg calcium | 350mg potassium | 80mg phosphorus | 1mg iron | 0mcg vitamin D

Vegetable and Chickpea Stew

Prep Time: 15 minutes | **Cooking Time:** 30 minutes | **Total Time:** 45 minutes | **Serving:** 4 | **Difficulty:** Easy

Ingredients:

- 2 cans (15 ounces each) chickpeas, drained and rinsed
- 1 medium carrot, diced
- 1 small zucchini, diced
- 1 small onion, chopped
- 2 cloves garlic, minced
- 1 tablespoon olive oil
- 4 cups low-sodium vegetable broth
- 1 teaspoon ground cumin
- 1 teaspoon ground coriander
- Salt and pepper, to taste
- Fresh cilantro, chopped (optional for garnish)

Instructions:

1. In a large pot, heat the olive oil over medium heat. Add the onion, garlic, carrot, and zucchini, sautéing until softened, about 5 minutes.
2. Add the chickpeas, vegetable broth, cumin, and coriander. Bring to a boil, then reduce the heat and simmer for 25-30 minutes, or until the vegetables are tender.
3. Season with salt and pepper to taste.
4. Serve hot, garnished with fresh cilantro if desired.

Nutritional Value:

300 calories | 8g fat | 1g saturated fat | 0mg cholesterol | 240mg sodium | 45g carbohydrate | 8g fiber | 6g sugar | 12g protein | 80mg calcium | 500mg potassium | 150mg phosphorus | 3mg iron | 0mcg vitamin D

Cream of Spinach Soup

Prep Time: 10 minutes | **Cooking Time:** 20 minutes | **Total Time:** 30 minutes | **Serving:** 4 | **Difficulty:** Easy

Ingredients:

- 6 cups fresh spinach leaves, washed and trimmed
- 1 medium onion, chopped
- 2 cloves garlic, minced
- 2 tablespoons unsalted butter
- 3 cups low-sodium vegetable broth
- 1 cup low-fat milk
- Salt and pepper, to taste
- Fresh nutmeg, grated (optional for garnish)

Instructions:

1. In a large pot, melt the butter over medium heat. Add the onion and

garlic, sautéing until softened, about 5 minutes.

2. Add the spinach and cook until wilted, about 3 minutes.

3. Add the vegetable broth and bring to a boil. Reduce the heat and simmer for 10 minutes.

4. Use an immersion blender to puree the soup until smooth, or transfer to a blender in batches.

5. Stir in the milk and season with salt and pepper to taste.

6. Simmer for an additional 5 minutes.

7. Serve hot, garnished with freshly grated nutmeg if desired.

Nutritional Value:

170 calories | 7g fat | 4g saturated fat | 15mg cholesterol | 220mg sodium | 18g carbohydrate | 3g fiber | 6g sugar | 5g protein | 120mg calcium | 400mg potassium | 80mg phosphorus | 2mg iron | 0mcg vitamin D

Vegetable and White Bean Soup

Prep Time: 15 minutes | **Cooking Time:** 30 minutes | **Total Time:** 45 minutes | **Serving:** 4 | **Difficulty:** Easy

Ingredients:

- 1 can (15 ounces) white beans, drained and rinsed
- 1 medium carrot, diced
- 1 celery stalk, diced
- 1 small zucchini, diced
- 1 small onion, chopped
- 2 cloves garlic, minced
- 1 tablespoon olive oil
- 4 cups low-sodium vegetable broth
- 1 teaspoon dried thyme
- Salt and pepper, to taste
- Fresh parsley, chopped (optional for garnish)

Instructions:

1. In a large pot, heat the olive oil over medium heat. Add the onion, garlic, carrot, and celery, sautéing until softened, about 5 minutes.

2. Add the white beans, zucchini, vegetable broth, and thyme. Bring to a boil, then reduce the heat and simmer for 25-30 minutes, or until the vegetables are tender.

3. Season with salt and pepper to taste.

4. Serve hot, garnished with fresh parsley if desired.

Nutritional Value:

210 calories | 5g fat | 1g saturated fat | 0mg cholesterol | 220mg sodium | 35g carbohydrate | 7g fiber | 5g sugar | 10g protein | 60mg calcium | 450mg potassium |

130mg phosphorus | 2mg iron | 0mcg vitamin D

Cream of Tomato Soup (No Seeds)

Prep Time: 10 minutes | **Cooking Time:** 20 minutes | **Total Time:** 30 minutes | **Serving:** 4 | **Difficulty:** Easy

Ingredients:

- 4 large tomatoes, peeled and seeded, chopped
- 1 medium onion, chopped
- 2 cloves garlic, minced
- 2 tablespoons unsalted butter
- 3 cups low-sodium vegetable broth
- 1 cup low-fat milk
- 1 tablespoon all-purpose flour
- 1 teaspoon sugar
- Salt and pepper, to taste
- Fresh basil, chopped (optional for garnish)

Instructions:

1. In a large pot, melt the butter over medium heat. Add the onion and garlic, sautéing until softened, about 5 minutes.
2. Stir in the flour and cook for 1-2 minutes, stirring constantly.
3. Add the chopped tomatoes, vegetable broth, and sugar. Bring to a boil, then reduce the heat and simmer for 15 minutes.
4. Use an immersion blender to puree the soup until smooth, or transfer to a blender in batches.
5. Stir in the milk and season with salt and pepper to taste.
6. Simmer for an additional 5 minutes.
7. Serve hot, garnished with fresh basil if desired.

Nutritional Value:

180 calories | 7g fat | 4g saturated fat | 15mg cholesterol | 220mg sodium | 25g carbohydrate | 3g fiber | 10g sugar | 4g protein | 120mg calcium | 400mg potassium | 90mg phosphorus | 1mg iron | 0mcg vitamin D

Vegetable and Orzo Soup

Prep Time: 10 minutes | **Cooking Time:** 20 minutes | **Total Time:** 30 minutes | **Serving:** 4 | **Difficulty:** Easy

Ingredients:

- 1/2 cup orzo pasta
- 1 medium carrot, diced
- 1 celery stalk, diced
- 1 small zucchini, diced

- 1 small onion, chopped

- 2 cloves garlic, minced

- 1 tablespoon olive oil

- 4 cups low-sodium vegetable broth

- 1 teaspoon dried oregano

- Salt and pepper, to taste

- Fresh parsley, chopped (optional for garnish)

Instructions:

1. In a large pot, heat the olive oil over medium heat. Add the onion, garlic, carrot, and celery, sautéing until softened, about 5 minutes.

2. Add the orzo, zucchini, vegetable broth, and oregano. Bring to a boil, then reduce the heat and simmer for 10-12 minutes, or until the orzo is tender.

3. Season with salt and pepper to taste.

4. Serve hot, garnished with fresh parsley if desired.

Nutritional Value:

200 calories | 5g fat | 1g saturated fat | 0mg cholesterol | 220mg sodium | 35g carbohydrate | 3g fiber | 4g sugar | 6g protein | 50mg calcium | 350mg potassium | 100mg phosphorus | 1mg iron | 0mcg vitamin D

Cream of Cucumber Soup

Prep Time: 10 minutes | **Cooking Time:** 10 minutes | **Total Time:** 20 minutes | **Serving:** 4 | **Difficulty:** Easy

Ingredients:

- 4 medium cucumbers, peeled, seeded, and chopped

- 1 small onion, chopped

- 2 cloves garlic, minced

- 2 tablespoons unsalted butter

- 2 cups low-sodium vegetable broth

- 1 cup low-fat yogurt

- 1 tablespoon fresh dill, chopped

- Salt and pepper, to taste

Instructions:

1. In a large pot, melt the butter over medium heat. Add the onion and garlic, sautéing until softened, about 5 minutes.

2. Add the chopped cucumbers and vegetable broth. Bring to a boil, then reduce the heat and simmer for 5 minutes.

3. Use an immersion blender to puree the soup until smooth, or transfer to a blender in batches.

4. Stir in the yogurt and dill, and season with salt and pepper to taste.

5. Simmer for an additional 5 minutes.

6. Serve hot, garnished with additional fresh dill if desired.

Nutritional Value:
150 calories | 6g fat | 3g saturated fat | 15mg cholesterol | 220mg sodium | 18g carbohydrate | 2g fiber | 6g sugar | 4g protein | 100mg calcium | 250mg potassium | 80mg phosphorus | 1mg iron | 0mcg vitamin D

Vegetable and Millet Soup

Prep Time: 10 minutes | **Cooking Time:** 30 minutes | **Total Time:** 40 minutes | **Serving:** 4 | **Difficulty:** Easy

Ingredients:

- 1/2 cup millet, rinsed
- 1 medium carrot, diced
- 1 celery stalk, diced
- 1 small zucchini, diced
- 1 small onion, chopped
- 2 cloves garlic, minced
- 1 tablespoon olive oil
- 4 cups low-sodium vegetable broth
- 1 teaspoon dried thyme
- Salt and pepper, to taste
- Fresh parsley, chopped (optional for garnish)

Instructions:

1. In a large pot, heat the olive oil over medium heat. Add the onion, garlic, carrot, and celery, sautéing until softened, about 5 minutes.

2. Add the millet, zucchini, vegetable broth, and thyme. Bring to a boil, then reduce the heat and simmer for 25-30 minutes, or until the millet is tender.

3. Season with salt and pepper to taste.

4. Serve hot, garnished with fresh parsley if desired.

Nutritional Value:
200 calories | 6g fat | 1g saturated fat | 0mg cholesterol | 220mg sodium | 35g carbohydrate | 4g fiber | 3g sugar | 5g protein | 50mg calcium | 350mg potassium | 100mg phosphorus | 1mg iron | 0mcg vitamin D

Cream of Fennel Soup

Prep Time: 10 minutes | **Cooking Time:** 20 minutes | **Total Time:** 30 minutes | **Serving:** 4 | **Difficulty:** Easy

Ingredients:

- 2 large fennel bulbs, trimmed and chopped
- 1 medium onion, chopped
- 2 cloves garlic, minced
- 2 tablespoons unsalted butter

- 3 cups low-sodium vegetable broth

- 1 cup low-fat milk

- Salt and pepper, to taste

- Fresh dill, chopped (optional for garnish)

Instructions:

1. In a large pot, melt the butter over medium heat. Add the onion, garlic, and fennel, sautéing until softened, about 8 minutes.

2. Add the vegetable broth and bring to a boil. Reduce the heat and simmer for 15 minutes, or until the fennel is tender.

3. Use an immersion blender to puree the soup until smooth, or transfer to a blender in batches.

4. Stir in the milk and season with salt and pepper to taste.

5. Simmer for an additional 5 minutes.

6. Serve hot, garnished with fresh dill if desired.

Nutritional Value:

180 calories | 8g fat | 4g saturated fat | 15mg cholesterol | 220mg sodium | 20g carbohydrate | 4g fiber | 8g sugar | 5g protein | 120mg calcium | 350mg potassium | 80mg phosphorus | 1mg iron | 0mcg vitamin D

Vegetable and Quinoa Soup

Prep Time: 10 minutes | **Cooking Time:** 25 minutes | **Total Time:** 35 minutes | **Serving:** 4 | **Difficulty:** Easy

Ingredients:

- 1/2 cup quinoa, rinsed

- 1 medium carrot, diced

- 1 celery stalk, diced

- 1 small zucchini, diced

- 1 small onion, chopped

- 2 cloves garlic, minced

- 1 tablespoon olive oil

- 4 cups low-sodium vegetable broth

- 1 teaspoon dried oregano

- Salt and pepper, to taste

- Fresh parsley, chopped (optional for garnish)

Instructions:

1. In a large pot, heat the olive oil over medium heat. Add the onion, garlic, carrot, and celery, sautéing until softened, about 5 minutes.

2. Add the quinoa, zucchini, vegetable broth, and oregano. Bring to a boil, then reduce the heat and simmer for 20-25 minutes, or until the quinoa is tender.

3. Season with salt and pepper to taste.

4. Serve hot, garnished with fresh parsley if desired.

Nutritional Value:
210 calories | 6g fat | 1g saturated fat | 0mg cholesterol | 220mg sodium | 35g carbohydrate | 5g fiber | 4g sugar | 6g protein | 50mg calcium | 350mg potassium | 100mg phosphorus | 1mg iron | 0mcg vitamin D

Cream of Parsnip Soup

Prep Time: 10 minutes | **Cooking Time:** 25 minutes | **Total Time:** 35 minutes | **Serving:** 4 | **Difficulty:** Easy

Ingredients:

- 4 large parsnips, peeled and chopped

- 1 medium onion, chopped

- 2 cloves garlic, minced

- 2 tablespoons unsalted butter

- 3 cups low-sodium vegetable broth

- 1 cup low-fat milk

- Salt and pepper, to taste

- Fresh chives, chopped (optional for garnish)

Instructions:

1. In a large pot, melt the butter over medium heat. Add the onion, garlic, and parsnips, sautéing until softened, about 8 minutes.

2. Add the vegetable broth and bring to a boil. Reduce the heat and simmer for 20 minutes, or until the parsnips are tender.

3. Use an immersion blender to puree the soup until smooth, or transfer to a blender in batches.

4. Stir in the milk and season with salt and pepper to taste.

5. Simmer for an additional 5 minutes.

6. Serve hot, garnished with fresh chives if desired.

Nutritional Value:
190 calories | 8g fat | 4g saturated fat | 15mg cholesterol | 220mg sodium | 25g carbohydrate | 6g fiber | 7g sugar | 5g protein | 120mg calcium | 400mg potassium | 80mg phosphorus | 1mg iron | 0mcg vitamin D

Vegetable and Farro Soup

Prep Time: 10 minutes | **Cooking Time:** 30 minutes | **Total Time:** 40 minutes | **Serving:** 4 | **Difficulty:** Easy

Ingredients:

- 1/2 cup farro, rinsed

- 1 medium carrot, diced

- 1 celery stalk, diced

- 1 small zucchini, diced

- 1 small onion, chopped

- 2 cloves garlic, minced

- 1 tablespoon olive oil

- 4 cups low-sodium vegetable broth

- 1 teaspoon dried thyme

- Salt and pepper, to taste

- Fresh parsley, chopped (optional for garnish)

Instructions:

1. In a large pot, heat the olive oil over medium heat. Add the onion, garlic, carrot, and celery, sautéing until softened, about 5 minutes.

2. Add the farro, zucchini, vegetable broth, and thyme. Bring to a boil, then reduce the heat and simmer for 25-30 minutes, or until the farro is tender.

3. Season with salt and pepper to taste.

4. Serve hot, garnished with fresh parsley if desired.

Nutritional Value:

220 calories | 6g fat | 1g saturated fat | 0mg cholesterol | 220mg sodium | 38g carbohydrate | 5g fiber | 4g sugar | 6g protein | 50mg calcium | 400mg potassium | 100mg phosphorus | 1mg iron | 0mcg vitamin D

Cream of Celeriac Soup

Prep Time: 10 minutes | **Cooking Time:** 25 minutes | **Total Time:** 35 minutes | **Serving:** 4 | **Difficulty:** Easy

Ingredients:

- 1 large celeriac (celery root), peeled and chopped

- 1 medium onion, chopped

- 2 cloves garlic, minced

- 2 tablespoons unsalted butter

- 3 cups low-sodium vegetable broth

- 1 cup low-fat milk

- Salt and pepper, to taste

- Fresh thyme, chopped (optional for garnish)

Instructions:

1. In a large pot, melt the butter over medium heat. Add the onion, garlic, and celeriac, sautéing until softened, about 8 minutes.

2. Add the vegetable broth and bring to a boil. Reduce the heat and simmer for 20 minutes, or until the celeriac is tender.

3. Use an immersion blender to puree the soup until smooth, or transfer to a blender in batches.

4. Stir in the milk and season with salt and pepper to taste.

5. Simmer for an additional 5 minutes.

6. Serve hot, garnished with fresh thyme if desired.

Nutritional Value:
180 calories | 8g fat | 4g saturated fat | 15mg cholesterol | 220mg sodium | 22g carbohydrate | 5g fiber | 6g sugar | 5g protein | 120mg calcium | 300mg potassium | 80mg phosphorus | 1mg iron | 0mcg vitamin D

Vegetable and Bulgur Soup

Prep Time: 10 minutes | **Cooking Time:** 25 minutes | **Total Time:** 35 minutes | **Serving:** 4 | **Difficulty:** Easy

Ingredients:

- 1/2 cup bulgur wheat, rinsed
- 1 medium carrot, diced
- 1 celery stalk, diced
- 1 small zucchini, diced
- 1 small onion, chopped
- 2 cloves garlic, minced
- 1 tablespoon olive oil
- 4 cups low-sodium vegetable broth
- 1 teaspoon dried basil
- Salt and pepper, to taste
- Fresh parsley, chopped (optional for garnish)

Instructions:

1. In a large pot, heat the olive oil over medium heat. Add the onion, garlic, carrot, and celery, sautéing until softened, about 5 minutes.

2. Add the bulgur, zucchini, vegetable broth, and basil. Bring to a boil, then reduce the heat and simmer for 20-25 minutes, or until the bulgur is tender.

3. Season with salt and pepper to taste.

4. Serve hot, garnished with fresh parsley if desired.

Nutritional Value:
200 calories | 6g fat | 1g saturated fat | 0mg cholesterol | 220mg sodium | 35g carbohydrate | 5g fiber | 4g sugar | 5g protein | 50mg calcium | 350mg potassium | 100mg phosphorus | 1mg iron | 0mcg vitamin D

Cream of Artichoke Soup

Prep Time: 10 minutes | **Cooking Time:** 25 minutes | **Total Time:** 35 minutes | **Serving:** 4 | **Difficulty:** Easy

Ingredients:

- 1 can (14 ounces) artichoke hearts, drained and chopped

60

- 1 medium onion, chopped

- 2 cloves garlic, minced

- 2 tablespoons unsalted butter

- 3 cups low-sodium vegetable broth

- 1 cup low-fat milk

- Salt and pepper, to taste

- Fresh parsley, chopped (optional for garnish)

Instructions:

1. In a large pot, melt the butter over medium heat. Add the onion, garlic, and artichoke hearts, sautéing until the onion is softened, about 8 minutes.

2. Add the vegetable broth and bring to a boil. Reduce the heat and simmer for 15 minutes.

3. Use an immersion blender to puree the soup until smooth, or transfer to a blender in batches.

4. Stir in the milk and season with salt and pepper to taste.

5. Simmer for an additional 5 minutes.

6. Serve hot, garnished with fresh parsley if desired.

Nutritional Value:
170 calories | 8g fat | 4g saturated fat | 15mg cholesterol | 220mg sodium | 18g carbohydrate | 4g fiber | 4g sugar | 5g protein | 120mg calcium | 300mg potassium

| 80mg phosphorus | 1mg iron | 0mcg vitamin D

Vegetable and Pearl Barley Soup

Prep Time: 10 minutes | **Cooking Time:** 30 minutes | **Total Time:** 40 minutes | **Serving:** 4 | **Difficulty:** Easy

Ingredients:

- 1/2 cup pearl barley, rinsed

- 1 medium carrot, diced

- 1 celery stalk, diced

- 1 small zucchini, diced

- 1 small onion, chopped

- 2 cloves garlic, minced

- 1 tablespoon olive oil

- 4 cups low-sodium vegetable broth

- 1 teaspoon dried thyme

- Salt and pepper, to taste

- Fresh parsley, chopped (optional for garnish)

Instructions:

1. In a large pot, heat the olive oil over medium heat. Add the onion, garlic, carrot, and celery, sautéing until softened, about 5 minutes.

2. Add the pearl barley, zucchini, vegetable broth, and thyme. Bring to

a boil, then reduce the heat and simmer for 25-30 minutes, or until the barley is tender.

3. Season with salt and pepper to taste.

4. Serve hot, garnished with fresh parsley if desired.

Nutritional Value:

220 calories | 6g fat | 1g saturated fat | 0mg cholesterol | 220mg sodium | 40g carbohydrate | 6g fiber | 4g sugar | 5g protein | 50mg calcium | 350mg potassium |

- 4 medium kohlrabi, peeled and diced

- 1 medium onion, chopped

- 2 cloves garlic, minced

- 2 tablespoons unsalted butter

Instructions:

1. In a large pot, melt the butter over medium heat. Add the onion, garlic, and kohlrabi, sautéing until softened, about 8 minutes.

2. Add the vegetable broth and bring to a boil. Reduce the heat and simmer for 15-20 minutes, or until the kohlrabi is tender.

3. Use an immersion blender to puree the soup until smooth, or transfer to a blender in batches.

100mg phosphorus | 1mg iron | 0mcg vitamin D

Cream of Kohlrabi Soup

Prep Time: 10 minutes | **Cooking Time:** 20 minutes | **Total Time:** 30 minutes | **Serving:** 4 | **Difficulty:** Easy

Ingredients:

- 3 cups low-sodium vegetable broth

- 1 cup low-fat milk

- Salt and pepper, to taste

- Fresh dill, chopped (optional for garnish)

4. Stir in the milk and season with salt and pepper to taste.

5. Simmer for an additional 5 minutes.

6. Serve hot, garnished with fresh dill if desired.

Nutritional Value:

170 calories | 8g fat | 4g saturated fat | 15mg cholesterol | 220mg sodium | 20g carbohydrate | 5g fiber | 6g sugar | 5g protein | 120mg calcium | 350mg potassium | 80mg phosphorus | 1mg iron | 0mcg vitamin D

Main Dishes

Baked Chicken Breast with Herbs

Prep Time: 10 minutes | **Cooking Time:** 25 minutes | **Total Time:** 35 minutes | **Serving:** 4 | **Difficulty:** Easy

Ingredients:

- 4 boneless, skinless chicken breasts
- 2 tablespoons olive oil
- 1 teaspoon dried thyme
- 1 teaspoon dried rosemary
- 1 teaspoon garlic powder
- Salt and pepper, to taste
- Fresh parsley, chopped (optional for garnish)

Instructions:

1. Preheat your oven to 375°F (190°C).
2. In a small bowl, mix together the olive oil, thyme, rosemary, garlic powder, salt, and pepper.
3. Rub the herb mixture evenly over the chicken breasts.
4. Place the chicken breasts in a baking dish and bake for 25-30 minutes, or until the chicken is cooked through and the internal temperature reaches 165°F (74°C).
5. Remove from the oven and let the chicken rest for 5 minutes before serving.
6. Serve hot, garnished with fresh parsley if desired.

Nutritional Value:

220 calories | 10g fat | 2g saturated fat | 75mg cholesterol | 240mg sodium | 0g carbohydrate | 0g fiber | 0g sugar | 26g protein | 20mg calcium | 300mg potassium | 220mg phosphorus | 1mg iron | 0mcg vitamin D

Grilled Salmon with Dill

Prep Time: 10 minutes | **Cooking Time:** 10 minutes | **Total Time:** 20 minutes | **Serving:** 4 | **Difficulty:** Easy

Ingredients:

- 4 salmon fillets (about 6 ounces each)
- 2 tablespoons olive oil
- 1 tablespoon fresh dill, chopped
- 1 clove garlic, minced
- Salt and pepper, to taste

- Lemon wedges for serving (optional)

Instructions:

1. Preheat your grill to medium-high heat.

2. In a small bowl, mix together the olive oil, dill, garlic, salt, and pepper.

3. Brush the salmon fillets with the olive oil mixture.

4. Place the salmon fillets on the grill, skin side down. Grill for 4-6 minutes on each side, or until the salmon is cooked to your desired doneness.

5. Remove from the grill and let rest for a few minutes before serving.

6. Serve hot, with lemon wedges on the side if desired.

Nutritional Value:

300 calories | 18g fat | 3g saturated fat | 70mg cholesterol | 150mg sodium | 0g carbohydrate | 0g fiber | 0g sugar | 32g protein | 20mg calcium | 500mg potassium | 250mg phosphorus | 1mg iron | 0mcg vitamin D

Steamed White Fish with Lemon

Prep Time: 5 minutes | **Cooking Time:** 10 minutes | **Total Time:** 15 minutes | **Serving:** 4 | **Difficulty:** Easy

Ingredients:

- 4 white fish fillets (such as cod or haddock)

- 2 tablespoons olive oil

- 1 lemon, thinly sliced

- 1 teaspoon garlic powder

- Salt and pepper, to taste

- Fresh parsley, chopped (optional for garnish)

Instructions:

1. Place the fish fillets in a steamer basket over boiling water.

2. Drizzle the olive oil over the fillets and sprinkle with garlic powder, salt, and pepper.

3. Top each fillet with a few slices of lemon.

4. Cover and steam for 8-10 minutes, or until the fish is opaque and flakes easily with a fork.

5. Serve hot, garnished with fresh parsley if desired.

Nutritional Value:

180 calories | 8g fat | 1g saturated fat | 60mg cholesterol | 220mg sodium | 2g carbohydrate | 1g fiber | 0g sugar | 24g protein | 20mg calcium | 400mg potassium | 200mg phosphorus | 1mg iron | 0mcg vitamin D

Chicken and Rice Casserole

Prep Time: 15 minutes | **Cooking Time:** 45 minutes | **Total Time:** 60 minutes | **Serving:** 6 | **Difficulty:** Easy

Ingredients:

- 2 cups cooked white rice
- 2 cups cooked chicken breast, shredded
- 1 cup low-sodium chicken broth
- 1 cup low-fat milk
- 1 cup frozen peas
- 1 small onion, finely chopped
- 2 cloves garlic, minced
- 2 tablespoons olive oil
- 1 teaspoon dried thyme
- 1 teaspoon dried parsley
- Salt and pepper, to taste

Instructions:

1. Preheat your oven to 350°F (175°C).
2. In a large skillet, heat the olive oil over medium heat. Add the onion and garlic, sautéing until softened, about 5 minutes.
3. In a large mixing bowl, combine the cooked rice, shredded chicken, sautéed onions and garlic, peas, thyme, parsley, salt, and pepper.
4. In a separate bowl, whisk together the chicken broth and milk. Pour over the rice mixture and stir until well combined.
5. Transfer the mixture to a lightly greased baking dish.
6. Bake for 30-35 minutes, or until the casserole is heated through and slightly golden on top.
7. Serve hot.

Nutritional Value:

280 calories | 8g fat | 2g saturated fat | 60mg cholesterol | 280mg sodium | 30g carbohydrate | 2g fiber | 3g sugar | 22g protein | 80mg calcium | 400mg potassium | 220mg phosphorus | 1.5mg iron | 0mcg vitamin D

Baked Tofu Squares

Prep Time: 10 minutes | **Cooking Time:** 25 minutes | **Total Time:** 35 minutes | **Serving:** 4 | **Difficulty:** Easy

Ingredients:

- 1 block (14 ounces) firm tofu, drained and pressed
- 2 tablespoons soy sauce (low-sodium)
- 1 tablespoon olive oil
- 1 teaspoon garlic powder
- 1 teaspoon ground ginger

- 1 teaspoon sesame oil (optional)

- Fresh scallions, chopped (optional for garnish)

Instructions:

1. Preheat your oven to 375°F (190°C).

2. Cut the tofu into 1-inch squares.

3. In a small bowl, mix together the soy sauce, olive oil, garlic powder, ground ginger, and sesame oil if using.

4. Toss the tofu squares in the marinade until well coated.

5. Arrange the tofu squares in a single layer on a parchment-lined baking sheet.

6. Bake for 20-25 minutes, flipping halfway through, until the tofu is golden and slightly crispy.

7. Serve hot, garnished with fresh scallions if desired.

Nutritional Value:

160 calories | 10g fat | 2g saturated fat | 0mg cholesterol | 320mg sodium | 4g carbohydrate | 1g fiber | 1g sugar | 14g protein | 150mg calcium | 300mg potassium | 150mg phosphorus | 2mg iron | 0mcg vitamin D

Spinach and Cheese Quiche

Prep Time: 15 minutes | **Cooking Time:** 35 minutes | **Total Time:** 50 minutes | **Serving:** 6 | **Difficulty:** Easy

Ingredients:

- 1 store-bought pie crust (or homemade)

- 4 large eggs

- 1 cup low-fat milk

- 1 cup fresh spinach, chopped

- 1/2 cup shredded low-fat cheese (such as cheddar or mozzarella)

- 1/4 cup finely chopped onion

- 1/4 teaspoon ground nutmeg

- Salt and pepper, to taste

Instructions:

1. Preheat your oven to 375°F (190°C).

2. In a medium mixing bowl, whisk together the eggs, milk, nutmeg, salt, and pepper.

3. Stir in the chopped spinach, shredded cheese, and chopped onion.

4. Pour the egg mixture into the pie crust.

5. Bake for 30-35 minutes, or until the quiche is set in the center and lightly golden on top.

6. Let cool for 5 minutes before slicing and serving.

Nutritional Value:
250 calories | 15g fat | 5g saturated fat | 160mg cholesterol | 320mg sodium | 16g carbohydrate | 1g fiber | 2g sugar | 12g protein | 150mg calcium | 300mg potassium | 200mg phosphorus | 2mg iron | 0.5mcg vitamin D

Baked Cod with Herbs

Prep Time: 10 minutes | **Cooking Time:** 15 minutes | **Total Time:** 25 minutes | **Serving:** 4 | **Difficulty:** Easy

Ingredients:

- 4 cod fillets (about 6 ounces each)
- 2 tablespoons olive oil
- 1 teaspoon dried thyme
- 1 teaspoon dried parsley
- 1 teaspoon garlic powder
- Salt and pepper, to taste
- Lemon wedges for serving (optional)

Instructions:

1. Preheat your oven to 400°F (200°C).
2. In a small bowl, mix together the olive oil, thyme, parsley, garlic powder, salt, and pepper.
3. Brush the herb mixture evenly over the cod fillets.

4. Place the fillets in a baking dish and bake for 12-15 minutes, or until the fish is opaque and flakes easily with a fork.
5. Serve hot, with lemon wedges on the side if desired.

Nutritional Value:
200 calories | 10g fat | 2g saturated fat | 60mg cholesterol | 220mg sodium | 0g carbohydrate | 0g fiber | 0g sugar | 24g protein | 20mg calcium | 400mg potassium | 200mg phosphorus | 1mg iron | 0mcg vitamin D

Grilled Chicken Skewers

Prep Time: 15 minutes | **Cooking Time:** 10 minutes | **Total Time:** 25 minutes | **Serving:** 4 | **Difficulty:** Easy

Ingredients:

- 1 pound chicken breast, cut into 1-inch cubes
- 2 tablespoons olive oil
- 1 teaspoon dried oregano
- 1 teaspoon garlic powder
- 1 teaspoon paprika
- Salt and pepper, to taste
- Wooden or metal skewers

Instructions:

1. If using wooden skewers, soak them in water for 30 minutes before grilling.

2. In a large bowl, toss the chicken cubes with olive oil, oregano, garlic powder, paprika, salt, and pepper until well coated.

3. Thread the chicken onto the skewers.

4. Preheat your grill to medium-high heat.

5. Grill the chicken skewers for 4-5 minutes on each side, or until the chicken is cooked through and has nice grill marks.

6. Serve hot.

Nutritional Value:

180 calories | 8g fat | 1g saturated fat | 70mg cholesterol | 220mg sodium | 0g carbohydrate | 0g fiber | 0g sugar | 26g protein | 20mg calcium | 300mg potassium | 200mg phosphorus | 1mg iron | 0mcg vitamin D

Poached Chicken Breast

Prep Time: 5 minutes | **Cooking Time:** 15 minutes | **Total Time:** 20 minutes | **Serving:** 4 | **Difficulty:** Easy

Ingredients:

- 4 boneless, skinless chicken breasts
- 4 cups low-sodium chicken broth
- 1 bay leaf
- 1 teaspoon dried thyme
- 2 cloves garlic, crushed
- Salt and pepper, to taste

Instructions:

1. In a large pot, combine the chicken broth, bay leaf, thyme, garlic, salt, and pepper. Bring to a simmer over medium heat.

2. Add the chicken breasts to the pot, making sure they are fully submerged in the broth.

3. Reduce the heat to low and cover the pot. Poach the chicken for 12-15 minutes, or until the chicken is cooked through and the internal temperature reaches 165°F (74°C).

4. Remove the chicken from the pot and let rest for a few minutes before slicing and serving.

5. Serve hot, with your choice of side dishes.

Nutritional Value:

150 calories | 4g fat | 1g saturated fat | 70mg cholesterol | 180mg sodium | 0g carbohydrate | 0g fiber | 0g sugar | 26g protein | 20mg calcium | 300mg potassium | 200mg phosphorus | 1mg iron | 0mcg vitamin D

Grilled Halibut

Prep Time: 10 minutes | **Cooking Time:** 10 minutes | **Total Time:** 20 minutes | **Serving:** 4 | **Difficulty:** Easy

Ingredients:

- 4 halibut fillets (about 6 ounces each)
- 2 tablespoons olive oil
- 1 tablespoon fresh dill, chopped
- 1 teaspoon garlic powder
- Salt and pepper, to taste
- Lemon wedges for serving (optional)

Instructions:

1. Preheat your grill to medium-high heat.
2. In a small bowl, mix together the olive oil, dill, garlic powder, salt, and pepper.
3. Brush the halibut fillets with the olive oil mixture.
4. Place the halibut fillets on the grill and cook for 4-5 minutes on each side, or until the fish is opaque and flakes easily with a fork.
5. Remove from the grill and let rest for a few minutes before serving.
6. Serve hot, with lemon wedges on the side if desired.

Nutritional Value:

230 calories | 11g fat | 2g saturated fat | 70mg cholesterol | 150mg sodium | 0g carbohydrate | 0g fiber | 0g sugar | 28g protein | 30mg calcium | 500mg potassium | 220mg phosphorus | 1mg iron | 0mcg vitamin D

Grilled Tofu Steaks

Prep Time: 10 minutes | **Cooking Time:** 15 minutes | **Total Time:** 25 minutes | **Serving:** 4 | **Difficulty:** Easy

Ingredients:

- 1 block (14 ounces) firm tofu, drained and pressed
- 2 tablespoons soy sauce (low-sodium)
- 1 tablespoon olive oil
- 1 teaspoon garlic powder
- 1 teaspoon ground ginger
- 1 teaspoon sesame oil (optional)
- Fresh scallions, chopped (optional for garnish)

Instructions:

1. Preheat your grill to medium heat.
2. Slice the tofu block into 4 thick steaks.
3. In a small bowl, mix together the soy sauce, olive oil, garlic powder,

ground ginger, and sesame oil if using.

4. Brush the tofu steaks with the marinade and let them sit for 10 minutes.

5. Place the tofu steaks on the grill and cook for 5-7 minutes on each side, or until they are lightly charred and heated through.

6. Serve hot, garnished with fresh scallions if desired.

Nutritional Value:

160 calories | 10g fat | 2g saturated fat | 0mg cholesterol | 320mg sodium | 4g carbohydrate | 1g fiber | 1g sugar | 14g protein | 150mg calcium | 300mg potassium | 150mg phosphorus | 2mg iron | 0mcg vitamin D

Baked Tilapia Fillet

Prep Time: 10 minutes | **Cooking Time:** 15 minutes | **Total Time:** 25 minutes | **Serving:** 4 | **Difficulty:** Easy

Ingredients:

- 4 tilapia fillets (about 6 ounces each)
- 2 tablespoons olive oil
- 1 teaspoon garlic powder
- 1 teaspoon dried thyme
- 1 teaspoon dried oregano
- Salt and pepper, to taste

- Lemon wedges for serving (optional)

Instructions:

1. Preheat your oven to 400°F (200°C).

2. In a small bowl, mix together the olive oil, garlic powder, thyme, oregano, salt, and pepper.

3. Brush the tilapia fillets with the olive oil mixture.

4. Place the fillets in a baking dish and bake for 12-15 minutes, or until the fish is opaque and flakes easily with a fork.

5. Serve hot, with lemon wedges on the side if desired.

Nutritional Value:

180 calories | 8g fat | 1g saturated fat | 60mg cholesterol | 220mg sodium | 0g carbohydrate | 0g fiber | 0g sugar | 24g protein | 20mg calcium | 400mg potassium | 200mg phosphorus | 1mg iron | 0mcg vitamin D

Baked Stuffed Bell Peppers

Prep Time: 20 minutes | **Cooking Time:** 40 minutes | **Total Time:** 60 minutes | **Serving:** 4 | **Difficulty:** Easy

Ingredients:

- 4 large bell peppers, tops cut off and seeds removed
- 1 cup cooked quinoa or rice

- 1 cup cooked ground chicken or turkey

- 1 small onion, chopped

- 2 cloves garlic, minced

- 1 cup shredded low-fat cheese (optional)

- 2 tablespoons olive oil

- 1 teaspoon dried oregano

- 1 teaspoon dried basil

- Salt and pepper, to taste

Instructions:

1. Preheat your oven to 375°F (190°C).

2. In a large skillet, heat the olive oil over medium heat. Add the onion and garlic, sautéing until softened, about 5 minutes.

3. Stir in the cooked quinoa or rice, cooked ground chicken or turkey, oregano, basil, salt, and pepper. Cook for an additional 2-3 minutes until well combined.

4. Stuff the bell peppers with the mixture and place them in a baking dish.

5. Cover the dish with foil and bake for 30 minutes.

6. Remove the foil and sprinkle the tops with cheese if using. Bake for an additional 10 minutes, or until the cheese is melted and bubbly.

7. Serve hot.

Nutritional Value:
250 calories | 10g fat | 3g saturated fat | 60mg cholesterol | 320mg sodium | 18g carbohydrate | 4g fiber | 6g sugar | 22g protein | 150mg calcium | 500mg potassium | 200mg phosphorus | 1.5mg iron | 0mcg vitamin D

Baked Salmon Fillet

Prep Time: 10 minutes | **Cooking Time:** 15 minutes | **Total Time:** 25 minutes | **Serving:** 4 | **Difficulty:** Easy

Ingredients:

- 4 salmon fillets (about 6 ounces each)

- 2 tablespoons olive oil

- 1 tablespoon fresh dill, chopped

- 1 teaspoon garlic powder

- Salt and pepper, to taste

- Lemon wedges for serving (optional)

Instructions:

1. Preheat your oven to 400°F (200°C).

2. In a small bowl, mix together the olive oil, dill, garlic powder, salt, and pepper.

3. Brush the salmon fillets with the olive oil mixture.

4. Place the fillets in a baking dish and bake for 12-15 minutes, or until the salmon is cooked to your desired doneness.

5. Serve hot, with lemon wedges on the side if desired.

Nutritional Value:

310 calories | 18g fat | 3g saturated fat | 70mg cholesterol | 150mg sodium | 0g carbohydrate | 0g fiber | 0g sugar | 34g protein | 20mg calcium | 500mg potassium | 250mg phosphorus | 1mg iron | 0mcg vitamin D

Baked Chicken Thighs

Prep Time: 10 minutes | **Cooking Time:** 35 minutes | **Total Time:** 45 minutes | **Serving:** 4 | **Difficulty:** Easy

Ingredients:

- 4 bone-in, skin-on chicken thighs
- 2 tablespoons olive oil
- 1 teaspoon garlic powder
- 1 teaspoon paprika
- 1 teaspoon dried thyme
- Salt and pepper, to taste

Instructions:

1. Preheat your oven to 400°F (200°C).

2. In a small bowl, mix together the olive oil, garlic powder, paprika, thyme, salt, and pepper.

3. Rub the seasoning mixture all over the chicken thighs.

4. Place the chicken thighs on a baking sheet, skin side up.

5. Bake for 35-40 minutes, or until the skin is crispy and the internal temperature reaches 165°F (74°C).

6. Serve hot.

Nutritional Value:

320 calories | 22g fat | 5g saturated fat | 90mg cholesterol | 240mg sodium | 0g carbohydrate | 0g fiber | 0g sugar | 28g protein | 20mg calcium | 300mg potassium | 200mg phosphorus | 1mg iron | 0mcg vitamin D

Baked Cod with Breadcrumbs

Prep Time: 10 minutes | **Cooking Time:** 15 minutes | **Total Time:** 25 minutes | **Serving:** 4 | **Difficulty:** Easy

Ingredients:

- 4 cod fillets (about 6 ounces each)
- 1/2 cup whole wheat breadcrumbs
- 2 tablespoons olive oil
- 1 teaspoon garlic powder
- 1 teaspoon dried parsley
- Salt and pepper, to taste
- Lemon wedges for serving (optional)

Instructions:

1. Preheat your oven to 400°F (200°C).

2. In a small bowl, mix together the breadcrumbs, olive oil, garlic powder, parsley, salt, and pepper.

3. Press the breadcrumb mixture onto the top of each cod fillet.

4. Place the fillets in a baking dish and bake for 12-15 minutes, or until the fish is opaque and flakes easily with a fork.

5. Serve hot, with lemon wedges on the side if desired.

Nutritional Value:
220 calories | 9g fat | 1g saturated fat | 60mg cholesterol | 220mg sodium | 10g carbohydrate | 1g fiber | 0g sugar | 26g protein | 20mg calcium | 400mg potassium | 200mg phosphorus | 1mg iron | 0mcg vitamin D

Steamed Mussels in White Wine

Prep Time: 10 minutes | **Cooking Time:** 10 minutes | **Total Time:** 20 minutes | **Serving:** 4 | **Difficulty:** Easy

Ingredients:

- 2 pounds mussels, cleaned and debearded
- 1 cup white wine
- 2 cloves garlic, minced
- 2 tablespoons unsalted butter
- 1 tablespoon fresh parsley, chopped
- Salt and pepper, to taste
- Lemon wedges for serving (optional)

Instructions:

1. In a large pot, melt the butter over medium heat. Add the garlic and sauté until fragrant, about 1 minute.

2. Add the white wine and bring to a simmer.

3. Add the mussels to the pot, cover, and steam for 5-7 minutes, or until the mussels have opened.

4. Discard any mussels that do not open.

5. Season with salt and pepper to taste, and stir in the fresh parsley.

6. Serve hot, with lemon wedges on the side if desired.

Nutritional Value:
190 calories | 8g fat | 4g saturated fat | 50mg cholesterol | 320mg sodium | 5g carbohydrate | 0g fiber | 0g sugar | 22g protein | 50mg calcium | 500mg potassium | 300mg phosphorus | 5mg iron | 0mcg vitamin D

Vegetable Side Dishes

Steamed Vegetable Medley

Prep Time: 10 minutes | **Cooking Time:** 10 minutes | **Total Time:** 20 minutes | **Serving:** 4 | **Difficulty:** Easy

Ingredients:

- 1 cup broccoli florets
- 1 cup cauliflower florets
- 1 cup sliced carrots
- 1 cup sliced zucchini
- 1 tablespoon olive oil
- Salt and pepper, to taste
- Fresh parsley, chopped (optional for garnish)

Instructions:

1. In a large pot, bring about 1 inch of water to a boil. Place a steamer basket in the pot.

2. Add the broccoli, cauliflower, carrots, and zucchini to the steamer basket.

3. Cover and steam the vegetables for 7-10 minutes, or until tender-crisp.

4. Transfer the steamed vegetables to a serving bowl and drizzle with olive oil.

5. Season with salt and pepper to taste, and garnish with fresh parsley if desired.

6. Serve hot.

Nutritional Value:

80 calories | 5g fat | 1g saturated fat | 0mg cholesterol | 40mg sodium | 8g carbohydrate | 3g fiber | 3g sugar | 2g protein | 30mg calcium | 250mg potassium | 60mg phosphorus | 1mg iron | 0mcg vitamin D

Steamed Broccoli with Olive Oil

Prep Time: 5 minutes | **Cooking Time:** 8 minutes | **Total Time:** 13 minutes | **Serving:** 4 | **Difficulty:** Easy

Ingredients:

- 4 cups broccoli florets
- 2 tablespoons olive oil
- Salt and pepper, to taste
- Lemon wedges for serving (optional)

Instructions:

1. In a large pot, bring about 1 inch of water to a boil. Place a steamer basket in the pot.

2. Add the broccoli florets to the steamer basket.

3. Cover and steam the broccoli for 5-8 minutes, or until tender-crisp.

4. Transfer the steamed broccoli to a serving bowl and drizzle with olive oil.

5. Season with salt and pepper to taste, and serve with lemon wedges if desired.

Nutritional Value:

70 calories | 5g fat | 1g saturated fat | 0mg cholesterol | 30mg sodium | 5g carbohydrate | 2g fiber | 2g sugar | 2g protein | 40mg calcium | 250mg potassium | 60mg phosphorus | 1mg iron | 0mcg vitamin D

Grilled Zucchini Slices

Prep Time: 10 minutes | **Cooking Time:** 6 minutes | **Total Time:** 16 minutes | **Serving:** 4 | **Difficulty:** Easy

Ingredients:

- 4 medium zucchinis, sliced into 1/4-inch rounds

- 2 tablespoons olive oil

- 1 teaspoon dried oregano

- Salt and pepper, to taste

Instructions:

1. Preheat your grill to medium-high heat.

2. In a large bowl, toss the zucchini slices with olive oil, oregano, salt, and pepper.

3. Place the zucchini slices on the grill and cook for 2-3 minutes on each side, or until grill marks appear and the zucchini is tender.

4. Serve hot.

Nutritional Value:

90 calories | 7g fat | 1g saturated fat | 0mg cholesterol | 40mg sodium | 6g carbohydrate | 2g fiber | 3g sugar | 2g protein | 30mg calcium | 300mg potassium | 60mg phosphorus | 1mg iron | 0mcg vitamin D

Steamed Asparagus with Lemon

Prep Time: 5 minutes | **Cooking Time:** 5 minutes | **Total Time:** 10 minutes | **Serving:** 4 | **Difficulty:** Easy

Ingredients:

- 1 pound asparagus, trimmed

- 2 tablespoons olive oil

- 1 tablespoon lemon juice

- Salt and pepper, to taste

Instructions:

1. In a large pot, bring about 1 inch of water to a boil. Place a steamer basket in the pot.

2. Add the asparagus to the steamer basket.

3. Cover and steam the asparagus for 4-5 minutes, or until tender-crisp.

4. Transfer the steamed asparagus to a serving bowl and drizzle with olive oil and lemon juice.

5. Season with salt and pepper to taste.

6. Serve hot.

Nutritional Value:
70 calories | 7g fat | 1g saturated fat | 0mg cholesterol | 30mg sodium | 4g carbohydrate | 2g fiber | 2g sugar | 2g protein | 30mg calcium | 200mg potassium | 60mg phosphorus | 1mg iron | 0mcg vitamin D

Steamed Green Beans

Prep Time: 5 minutes | **Cooking Time:** 8 minutes | **Total Time:** 13 minutes | **Serving:** 4 | **Difficulty:** Easy

Ingredients:

- 4 cups green beans, trimmed
- 2 tablespoons olive oil
- Salt and pepper, to taste
- Fresh dill, chopped (optional for garnish)

Instructions:

1. In a large pot, bring about 1 inch of water to a boil. Place a steamer basket in the pot.

2. Add the green beans to the steamer basket.

3. Cover and steam the green beans for 6-8 minutes, or until tender-crisp.

4. Transfer the steamed green beans to a serving bowl and drizzle with olive oil.

5. Season with salt and pepper to taste, and garnish with fresh dill if desired.

6. Serve hot.

Nutritional Value:
70 calories | 5g fat | 1g saturated fat | 0mg cholesterol | 30mg sodium | 7g carbohydrate | 3g fiber | 3g sugar | 2g protein | 40mg calcium | 250mg potassium | 60mg phosphorus | 1mg iron | 0mcg vitamin D

Baked Potato with Sour Cream

Prep Time: 5 minutes | **Cooking Time:** 50 minutes | **Total Time:** 55 minutes | **Serving:** 4 | **Difficulty:** Easy

Ingredients:

- 4 large russet potatoes
- 1/2 cup low-fat sour cream
- 2 tablespoons chives, chopped

- Salt and pepper, to taste

Instructions:

1. Preheat your oven to 400°F (200°C).

2. Scrub the potatoes clean and pierce them several times with a fork.

3. Place the potatoes directly on the oven rack and bake for 45-50 minutes, or until tender when pierced with a fork.

4. Remove the potatoes from the oven and let cool slightly before slicing them open.

5. Top each potato with a dollop of sour cream and a sprinkle of chopped chives.

6. Season with salt and pepper to taste.

7. Serve hot.

Nutritional Value:

200 calories | 3g fat | 1g saturated fat | 10mg cholesterol | 30mg sodium | 40g carbohydrate | 4g fiber | 2g sugar | 5g protein | 50mg calcium | 700mg potassium | 90mg phosphorus | 2mg iron | 0mcg vitamin D

Steamed Cauliflower with Butter

Prep Time: 5 minutes | **Cooking Time:** 10 minutes | **Total Time:** 15 minutes | **Serving:** 4 | **Difficulty:** Easy

Ingredients:

- 1 medium head of cauliflower, cut into florets

- 2 tablespoons unsalted butter, melted

- Salt and pepper, to taste

- Fresh parsley, chopped (optional for garnish)

Instructions:

1. In a large pot, bring about 1 inch of water to a boil. Place a steamer basket in the pot.

2. Add the cauliflower florets to the steamer basket.

3. Cover and steam the cauliflower for 8-10 minutes, or until tender.

4. Transfer the steamed cauliflower to a serving bowl and drizzle with melted butter.

5. Season with salt and pepper to taste, and garnish with fresh parsley if desired.

6. Serve hot.

Nutritional Value:

90 calories | 7g fat | 4g saturated fat | 20mg cholesterol | 40mg sodium | 5g carbohydrate | 2g fiber | 2g sugar | 2g protein | 30mg calcium | 200mg potassium | 60mg phosphorus | 1mg iron | 0mcg vitamin D

Baked Pumpkin Wedges

Prep Time: 10 minutes | **Cooking Time:** 25 minutes | **Total Time:** 35 minutes | **Serving:** 4 | **Difficulty:** Easy

Ingredients:

- 1 small pumpkin, peeled and cut into wedges
- 2 tablespoons olive oil
- 1 teaspoon ground cinnamon
- 1/4 teaspoon ground nutmeg (optional)
- Salt and pepper, to taste

Instructions:

1. Preheat your oven to 400°F (200°C).
2. In a large bowl, toss the pumpkin wedges with olive oil, cinnamon, nutmeg (if using), salt, and pepper.
3. Arrange the pumpkin wedges in a single layer on a baking sheet.
4. Bake for 20-25 minutes, or until the pumpkin is tender and lightly browned.
5. Serve hot.

Nutritional Value:
120 calories | 7g fat | 1g saturated fat | 0mg cholesterol | 60mg sodium | 14g carbohydrate | 3g fiber | 4g sugar | 2g protein | 40mg calcium | 400mg potassium | 80mg phosphorus | 1mg iron | 0mcg vitamin D

Steamed Brussels Sprouts

Prep Time: 5 minutes | **Cooking Time:** 8 minutes | **Total Time:** 13 minutes | **Serving:** 4 | **Difficulty:** Easy

Ingredients:

- 4 cups Brussels sprouts, trimmed and halved
- 2 tablespoons olive oil
- Salt and pepper, to taste

Instructions:

1. In a large pot, bring about 1 inch of water to a boil. Place a steamer basket in the pot.
2. Add the Brussels sprouts to the steamer basket.
3. Cover and steam the Brussels sprouts for 6-8 minutes, or until tender.
4. Transfer the steamed Brussels sprouts to a serving bowl and drizzle with olive oil.
5. Season with salt and pepper to taste.
6. Serve hot.

Nutritional Value:
80 calories | 5g fat | 1g saturated fat | 0mg

cholesterol | 40mg sodium | 7g carbohydrate | 3g fiber | 2g sugar | 3g protein | 40mg calcium | 350mg potassium | 60mg phosphorus | 1mg iron | 0mcg vitamin D

Steamed Artichoke with Butter

Prep Time: 10 minutes | **Cooking Time:** 30 minutes | **Total Time:** 40 minutes | **Serving:** 4 | **Difficulty:** Easy

Ingredients:

- 4 large artichokes, trimmed
- 1/4 cup unsalted butter, melted
- 1 tablespoon lemon juice
- Salt and pepper, to taste

Instructions:

1. Fill a large pot with about 2 inches of water and bring to a boil. Place a steamer basket in the pot.
2. Trim the artichokes by cutting off the top inch and removing the tough outer leaves.
3. Place the artichokes in the steamer basket, stem side up.
4. Cover and steam the artichokes for 25-30 minutes, or until the outer leaves can be easily pulled off.
5. In a small bowl, combine the melted butter and lemon juice.
6. Serve the artichokes hot, with the butter mixture on the side for dipping.

Nutritional Value:
150 calories | 12g fat | 7g saturated fat | 30mg cholesterol | 80mg sodium | 10g carbohydrate | 5g fiber | 1g sugar | 3g protein | 50mg calcium | 350mg potassium | 60mg phosphorus | 1mg iron | 0mcg vitamin D

Grilled Portobello Mushroom

Prep Time: 10 minutes | **Cooking Time:** 10 minutes | **Total Time:** 20 minutes | **Serving:** 4 | **Difficulty:** Easy

Ingredients:

- 4 large Portobello mushrooms, stems removed
- 2 tablespoons olive oil
- 1 tablespoon balsamic vinegar (optional, for those who can tolerate it)
- 1 teaspoon garlic powder
- 1 teaspoon dried thyme
- Salt and pepper, to taste

Instructions:

1. Preheat your grill to medium heat.
2. In a small bowl, mix together the olive oil, balsamic vinegar (if using),

garlic powder, thyme, salt, and pepper.

3. Brush the Portobello mushrooms with the mixture, coating both sides.

4. Place the mushrooms on the grill, gill side down, and cook for 5 minutes.

5. Flip the mushrooms and cook for an additional 5 minutes, or until tender.

6. Serve hot.

Nutritional Value:
90 calories | 7g fat | 1g saturated fat | 0mg cholesterol | 70mg sodium | 5g carbohydrate | 1g fiber | 2g sugar | 2g protein | 20mg calcium | 300mg potassium | 40mg phosphorus | 1mg iron | 0mcg vitamin D

Steamed Corn on the Cob

Prep Time: 5 minutes | **Cooking Time:** 10 minutes | **Total Time:** 15 minutes | **Serving:** 4 | **Difficulty:** Easy

Ingredients:

- 4 ears of corn, husked
- 2 tablespoons unsalted butter, melted
- Salt and pepper, to taste

Instructions:

1. In a large pot, bring about 1 inch of water to a boil. Place a steamer basket in the pot.

2. Add the ears of corn to the steamer basket.

3. Cover and steam the corn for 8-10 minutes, or until tender.

4. Transfer the steamed corn to a serving dish and brush with melted butter.

5. Season with salt and pepper to taste.

6. Serve hot.

Nutritional Value:
130 calories | 5g fat | 3g saturated fat | 10mg cholesterol | 20mg sodium | 24g carbohydrate | 2g fiber | 6g sugar | 3g protein | 0mg calcium | 270mg potassium | 0mg phosphorus | 1mg iron | 0mcg vitamin D

Steamed Bok Choy

Prep Time: 5 minutes | **Cooking Time:** 5 minutes | **Total Time:** 10 minutes | **Serving:** 4 | **Difficulty:** Easy

Ingredients:

- 4 cups baby bok choy, halved lengthwise
- 2 tablespoons olive oil
- 1 teaspoon sesame oil (optional)
- 2 cloves garlic, minced

- Salt and pepper, to taste

Instructions:

1. In a large pot, bring about 1 inch of water to a boil. Place a steamer basket in the pot.

2. Add the bok choy to the steamer basket.

3. Cover and steam the bok choy for 4-5 minutes, or until tender.

4. In a small saucepan, heat the olive oil and sesame oil (if using) over medium heat. Add the minced garlic and sauté until fragrant, about 1 minute.

5. Drizzle the garlic oil over the steamed bok choy.

6. Season with salt and pepper to taste.

7. Serve hot.

Nutritional Value:
70 calories | 5g fat | 1g saturated fat | 0mg cholesterol | 40mg sodium | 5g carbohydrate | 2g fiber | 2g sugar | 2g protein | 80mg calcium | 300mg potassium | 60mg phosphorus | 1mg iron | 0mcg vitamin D

Steamed Snow Peas

Prep Time: 5 minutes | **Cooking Time:** 5 minutes | **Total Time:** 10 minutes | **Serving:** 4 | **Difficulty:** Easy

Ingredients:

- 4 cups snow peas, trimmed
- 2 tablespoons olive oil
- Salt and pepper, to taste
- Fresh lemon zest (optional)

Instructions:

1. In a large pot, bring about 1 inch of water to a boil. Place a steamer basket in the pot.

2. Add the snow peas to the steamer basket.

3. Cover and steam the snow peas for 3-5 minutes, or until tender-crisp.

4. Transfer the steamed snow peas to a serving bowl and drizzle with olive oil.

5. Season with salt and pepper to taste, and garnish with fresh lemon zest if desired.

6. Serve hot.

Nutritional Value:
60 calories | 4g fat | 1g saturated fat | 0mg cholesterol | 20mg sodium | 5g carbohydrate | 2g fiber | 2g sugar | 2g protein | 20mg calcium | 180mg potassium | 40mg phosphorus | 1mg iron | 0mcg vitamin D

Grilled Eggplant Rounds

Prep Time: 10 minutes | **Cooking Time:** 10 minutes | **Total Time:** 20 minutes | **Serving:** 4 | **Difficulty:** Easy

Ingredients:

- 1 large eggplant, sliced into 1/2-inch rounds
- 2 tablespoons olive oil
- 1 teaspoon garlic powder
- 1 teaspoon dried oregano
- Salt and pepper, to taste

Instructions:

1. Preheat your grill to medium-high heat.
2. In a large bowl, toss the eggplant slices with olive oil, garlic powder, oregano, salt, and pepper.
3. Place the eggplant slices on the grill and cook for 4-5 minutes on each side, or until grill marks appear and the eggplant is tender.
4. Serve hot.

Nutritional Value:

80 calories | 5g fat | 1g saturated fat | 0mg cholesterol | 50mg sodium | 10g carbohydrate | 4g fiber | 3g sugar | 1g protein | 10mg calcium | 250mg potassium | 40mg phosphorus | 1mg iron | 0mcg vitamin D

Steamed Spinach with Garlic

Prep Time: 5 minutes | **Cooking Time:** 5 minutes | **Total Time:** 10 minutes | **Serving:** 4 | **Difficulty:** Easy

Ingredients:

- 8 cups fresh spinach leaves, washed and trimmed
- 2 tablespoons olive oil
- 2 cloves garlic, minced
- Salt and pepper, to taste

Instructions:

1. In a large pot, bring about 1 inch of water to a boil. Place a steamer basket in the pot.
2. Add the spinach to the steamer basket.
3. Cover and steam the spinach for 3-5 minutes, or until wilted.
4. In a small saucepan, heat the olive oil over medium heat. Add the minced garlic and sauté until fragrant, about 1 minute.
5. Drizzle the garlic oil over the steamed spinach.
6. Season with salt and pepper to taste.
7. Serve hot.

Nutritional Value:

80 calories | 5g fat | 1g saturated fat | 0mg

cholesterol | 50mg sodium | 7g carbohydrate | 4g fiber | 0g sugar | 2g protein | 80mg calcium | 500mg potassium | 40mg phosphorus | 2mg iron | 0mcg vitamin D

carbohydrate | 2g fiber | 2g sugar | 2g protein | 30mg calcium | 200mg potassium | 60mg phosphorus | 1mg iron | 0mcg vitamin D

Grilled Asparagus Spears

Prep Time: 5 minutes | **Cooking Time:** 8 minutes | **Total Time:** 13 minutes | **Serving:** 4 | **Difficulty:** Easy

Ingredients:

- 1 pound asparagus, trimmed
- 2 tablespoons olive oil
- Salt and pepper, to taste
- Fresh lemon juice (optional)

Instructions:

1. Preheat your grill to medium-high heat.
2. In a large bowl, toss the asparagus spears with olive oil, salt, and pepper.
3. Place the asparagus spears on the grill and cook for 3-4 minutes on each side, or until they are tender and slightly charred.
4. Serve hot, with a squeeze of fresh lemon juice if desired.

Nutritional Value:

70 calories | 5g fat | 1g saturated fat | 0mg cholesterol | 30mg sodium | 5g

Steamed Kale with Lemon

Prep Time: 5 minutes | **Cooking Time:** 8 minutes | **Total Time:** 13 minutes | **Serving:** 4 | **Difficulty:** Easy

Ingredients:

- 8 cups kale, washed and trimmed
- 2 tablespoons olive oil
- 1 tablespoon lemon juice
- Salt and pepper, to taste

Instructions:

1. In a large pot, bring about 1 inch of water to a boil. Place a steamer basket in the pot.
2. Add the kale to the steamer basket.
3. Cover and steam the kale for 5-8 minutes, or until tender.
4. Transfer the steamed kale to a serving bowl and drizzle with olive oil and lemon juice.
5. Season with salt and pepper to taste.
6. Serve hot.

Nutritional Value:

80 calories | 5g fat | 1g saturated fat | 0mg

cholesterol | 50mg sodium | 7g carbohydrate | 2g fiber | 1g sugar | 3g protein | 80mg calcium | 400mg potassium | 40mg phosphorus | 1mg iron | 0mcg vitamin D

Grilled Zucchini and Squash

Prep Time: 10 minutes | **Cooking Time:** 10 minutes | **Total Time:** 20 minutes | **Serving:** 4 | **Difficulty:** Easy

Ingredients:

- 2 medium zucchinis, sliced into rounds
- 2 medium yellow squashes, sliced into rounds
- 2 tablespoons olive oil
- 1 teaspoon garlic powder
- 1 teaspoon dried oregano
- Salt and pepper, to taste

Instructions:

1. Preheat your grill to medium-high heat.
2. In a large bowl, toss the zucchini and squash rounds with olive oil, garlic powder, oregano, salt, and pepper.
3. Place the zucchini and squash rounds on the grill and cook for 4-5 minutes on each side, or until grill marks appear and the vegetables are tender.

4. Serve hot.

Nutritional Value:

90 calories | 7g fat | 1g saturated fat | 0mg cholesterol | 50mg sodium | 6g carbohydrate | 2g fiber | 3g sugar | 2g protein | 30mg calcium | 300mg potassium | 60mg phosphorus | 1mg iron | 0mcg vitamin D

Steamed Cabbage Wedges

Prep Time: 5 minutes | **Cooking Time:** 10 minutes | **Total Time:** 15 minutes | **Serving:** 4 | **Difficulty:** Easy

Ingredients:

- 1 medium head of cabbage, cut into wedges
- 2 tablespoons unsalted butter, melted
- Salt and pepper, to taste

Instructions:

1. In a large pot, bring about 1 inch of water to a boil. Place a steamer basket in the pot.
2. Add the cabbage wedges to the steamer basket.
3. Cover and steam the cabbage for 8-10 minutes, or until tender.

4. Transfer the steamed cabbage to a serving dish and drizzle with melted butter.

5. Season with salt and pepper to taste.

6. Serve hot.

Nutritional Value:

90 calories | 7g fat | 4g saturated fat | 20mg cholesterol | 40mg sodium | 5g carbohydrate | 2g fiber | 3g sugar | 2g protein | 30mg calcium | 200mg potassium | 60mg phosphorus | 1mg iron | 0mcg vitamin D

Steamed Baby Carrots

Prep Time: 5 minutes | **Cooking Time:** 10 minutes | **Total Time:** 15 minutes | **Serving:** 4 | **Difficulty:** Easy

Ingredients:

- 4 cups baby carrots

- 2 tablespoons unsalted butter, melted

- Salt and pepper, to taste

- Fresh parsley, chopped (optional for garnish)

Instructions:

1. In a large pot, bring about 1 inch of water to a boil. Place a steamer basket in the pot.

2. Add the baby carrots to the steamer basket.

3. Cover and steam the carrots for 8-10 minutes, or until tender.

4. Transfer the steamed carrots to a serving bowl and drizzle with melted butter.

5. Season with salt and pepper to taste, and garnish with fresh parsley if desired.

6. Serve hot.

Nutritional Value:

80 calories | 5g fat | 3g saturated fat | 15mg cholesterol | 60mg sodium | 8g carbohydrate | 3g fiber | 5g sugar | 1g protein | 30mg calcium | 270mg potassium | 40mg phosphorus | 0.5mg iron | 0mcg vitamin D

Grilled Romaine Hearts

Prep Time: 5 minutes | **Cooking Time:** 5 minutes | **Total Time:** 10 minutes | **Serving:** 4 | **Difficulty:** Easy

Ingredients:

- 2 large romaine hearts, halved lengthwise

- 2 tablespoons olive oil

- Salt and pepper, to taste

- Lemon wedges for serving (optional)

Instructions:

1. Preheat your grill to medium-high heat.

2. Brush the cut sides of the romaine hearts with olive oil.

3. Place the romaine hearts on the grill, cut side down, and grill for 2-3 minutes until lightly charred and slightly wilted.

4. Remove from the grill, season with salt and pepper, and serve with lemon wedges if desired.

5. Serve warm.

Nutritional Value:

70 calories | 5g fat | 1g saturated fat | 0mg cholesterol | 30mg sodium | 4g carbohydrate | 2g fiber | 2g sugar | 1g protein | 20mg calcium | 150mg potassium | 30mg phosphorus | 0.5mg iron | 0mcg vitamin D

Steamed Swiss Chard

Prep Time: 5 minutes | **Cooking Time:** 8 minutes | **Total Time:** 13 minutes | **Serving:** 4 | **Difficulty:** Easy

Ingredients:

- 8 cups Swiss chard, washed and chopped
- 2 tablespoons olive oil
- 2 cloves garlic, minced
- Salt and pepper, to taste

Instructions:

1. In a large pot, bring about 1 inch of water to a boil. Place a steamer basket in the pot.

2. Add the chopped Swiss chard to the steamer basket.

3. Cover and steam the Swiss chard for 6-8 minutes, or until wilted and tender.

4. In a small saucepan, heat the olive oil over medium heat. Add the minced garlic and sauté until fragrant, about 1 minute.

5. Drizzle the garlic oil over the steamed Swiss chard.

6. Season with salt and pepper to taste.

7. Serve hot.

Nutritional Value:

80 calories | 5g fat | 1g saturated fat | 0mg cholesterol | 60mg sodium | 7g carbohydrate | 4g fiber | 1g sugar | 3g protein | 80mg calcium | 600mg potassium | 40mg phosphorus | 2mg iron | 0mcg vitamin D

Grilled Polenta Squares

Prep Time: 10 minutes | **Cooking Time:** 10 minutes | **Total Time:** 20 minutes | **Serving:** 4 | **Difficulty:** Easy

Ingredients:

- 1 tube (18 ounces) pre-cooked polenta, cut into 1/2-inch thick squares

- 2 tablespoons olive oil

- 1 teaspoon dried oregano

- Salt and pepper, to taste

- Fresh parsley, chopped (optional for garnish)

Instructions:

1. Preheat your grill to medium-high heat.

2. Brush the polenta squares with olive oil and season with oregano, salt, and pepper.

3. Place the polenta squares on the grill and cook for 4-5 minutes on each side, or until grill marks appear and the polenta is heated through.

4. Serve hot, garnished with fresh parsley if desired.

Nutritional Value:

150 calories | 8g fat | 1g saturated fat | 0mg cholesterol | 250mg sodium | 15g carbohydrate | 2g fiber | 1g sugar | 2g protein | 20mg calcium | 60mg potassium | 60mg phosphorus | 1mg iron | 0mcg vitamin D

Steamed Baby Potatoes

Prep Time: 5 minutes | **Cooking Time:** 15 minutes | **Total Time:** 20 minutes | **Serving:** 4 | **Difficulty:** Easy

Ingredients:

- 1 pound baby potatoes, washed

- 2 tablespoons unsalted butter, melted

- Salt and pepper, to taste

- Fresh dill, chopped (optional for garnish)

Instructions:

1. In a large pot, bring about 1 inch of water to a boil. Place a steamer basket in the pot.

2. Add the baby potatoes to the steamer basket.

3. Cover and steam the potatoes for 15 minutes, or until tender when pierced with a fork.

4. Transfer the steamed potatoes to a serving bowl and drizzle with melted butter.

5. Season with salt and pepper to taste, and garnish with fresh dill if desired.

6. Serve hot.

Nutritional Value:

130 calories | 4g fat | 2g saturated fat | 10mg cholesterol | 30mg sodium | 22g

carbohydrate | 3g fiber | 1g sugar | 2g protein | 20mg calcium | 450mg potassium | 60mg phosphorus | 1mg iron | 0mcg vitamin D

Steamed Edamame

Prep Time: 5 minutes | **Cooking Time:** 5 minutes | **Total Time:** 10 minutes | **Serving:** 4 | **Difficulty:** Easy

Ingredients:

- 4 cups frozen edamame (in pods)
- Salt, to taste

Instructions:

1. In a large pot, bring about 1 inch of water to a boil. Place a steamer basket in the pot.
2. Add the frozen edamame to the steamer basket.
3. Cover and steam the edamame for 4-5 minutes, or until heated through.
4. Transfer the steamed edamame to a serving bowl and sprinkle with salt to taste.
5. Serve hot.

Nutritional Value:
120 calories | 4g fat | 0.5g saturated fat | 0mg cholesterol | 30mg sodium | 9g carbohydrate | 4g fiber | 1g sugar | 11g protein | 60mg calcium | 400mg potassium | 160mg phosphorus | 2mg iron | 0mcg vitamin D

Steamed New Potatoes

Prep Time: 5 minutes | **Cooking Time:** 20 minutes | **Total Time:** 25 minutes | **Serving:** 4 | **Difficulty:** Easy

Ingredients:

- 1 pound new potatoes, washed
- 2 tablespoons olive oil
- 1 teaspoon dried rosemary
- Salt and pepper, to taste

Instructions:

1. In a large pot, bring about 1 inch of water to a boil. Place a steamer basket in the pot.
2. Add the new potatoes to the steamer basket.
3. Cover and steam the potatoes for 20 minutes, or until tender when pierced with a fork.
4. Transfer the steamed potatoes to a serving bowl and drizzle with olive oil.
5. Season with rosemary, salt, and pepper to taste.
6. Serve hot.

Nutritional Value:
130 calories | 4g fat | 0.5g saturated fat | 0mg cholesterol | 30mg sodium | 22g carbohydrate | 3g fiber | 1g sugar | 2g protein | 20mg calcium | 450mg potassium |

60mg phosphorus | 1mg iron | 0mcg vitamin D

Steamed Broccoli Rabe

Prep Time: 5 minutes | **Cooking Time:** 6 minutes | **Total Time:** 11 minutes | **Serving:** 4 | **Difficulty:** Easy

Ingredients:

- 1 bunch broccoli rabe, washed and trimmed
- 2 tablespoons olive oil
- 2 cloves garlic, minced
- Salt and pepper, to taste

Instructions:

1. In a large pot, bring about 1 inch of water to a boil. Place a steamer basket in the pot.
2. Add the broccoli rabe to the steamer basket.
3. Cover and steam the broccoli rabe for 5-6 minutes, or until tender.
4. In a small saucepan, heat the olive oil over medium heat. Add the minced garlic and sauté until fragrant, about 1 minute.
5. Drizzle the garlic oil over the steamed broccoli rabe.
6. Season with salt and pepper to taste.
7. Serve hot.

Nutritional Value:

70 calories | 5g fat | 1g saturated fat | 0mg cholesterol | 60mg sodium | 5g carbohydrate | 2g fiber | 1g sugar | 2g protein | 80mg calcium | 500mg potassium | 40mg phosphorus | 2mg iron | 0mcg vitamin D

Grilled Endive

Prep Time: 5 minutes | **Cooking Time:** 8 minutes | **Total Time:** 13 minutes | **Serving:** 4 | **Difficulty:** Easy

Ingredients:

- 4 heads Belgian endive, halved lengthwise
- 2 tablespoons olive oil
- Salt and pepper, to taste
- Balsamic vinegar (optional, for those who can tolerate it)

Instructions:

1. Preheat your grill to medium-high heat.
2. Brush the cut sides of the endive with olive oil.
3. Place the endive on the grill, cut side down, and grill for 3-4 minutes until slightly charred and tender.
4. Remove from the grill, season with salt and pepper, and drizzle with balsamic vinegar if using.
5. Serve warm.

Nutritional Value:

60 calories | 5g fat | 0.5g saturated fat | 0mg cholesterol | 20mg sodium | 4g carbohydrate | 2g fiber | 1g sugar | 1g protein | 40mg calcium | 200mg potassium | 40mg phosphorus | 0.5mg iron | 0mcg vitamin D

Steamed Sugar Snap Peas

Prep Time: 5 minutes | **Cooking Time:** 5 minutes | **Total Time:** 10 minutes | **Serving:** 4 | **Difficulty:** Easy

Ingredients:

- 4 cups sugar snap peas, trimmed
- 2 tablespoons olive oil
- Salt and pepper, to taste

Instructions:

1. In a large pot, bring about 1 inch of water to a boil. Place a steamer basket in the pot.
2. Add the sugar snap peas to the steamer basket.
3. Cover and steam the sugar snap peas for 4-5 minutes, or until tender-crisp.
4. Transfer the steamed sugar snap peas to a serving bowl and drizzle with olive oil.
5. Season with salt and pepper to taste.

6. Serve hot.

Nutritional Value:

70 calories | 5g fat | 1g saturated fat | 0mg cholesterol | 20mg sodium | 6g carbohydrate | 2g fiber | 3g sugar | 2g protein | 40mg calcium | 180mg potassium | 40mg phosphorus | 1mg iron | 0mcg vitamin D

Steamed Beet Wedges

Prep Time: 10 minutes | **Cooking Time:** 20 minutes | **Total Time:** 30 minutes | **Serving:** 4 | **Difficulty:** Easy

Ingredients:

- 4 medium beets, peeled and cut into wedges
- 2 tablespoons olive oil
- Salt and pepper, to taste
- Fresh dill, chopped (optional for garnish)

Instructions:

1. In a large pot, bring about 1 inch of water to a boil. Place a steamer basket in the pot.
2. Add the beet wedges to the steamer basket.
3. Cover and steam the beets for 15-20 minutes, or until tender when pierced with a fork.

4. Transfer the steamed beets to a serving bowl and drizzle with olive oil.

5. Season with salt and pepper to taste, and garnish with fresh dill if desired.

6. Serve warm.

Nutritional Value:
100 calories | 7g fat | 1g saturated fat | 0mg cholesterol | 60mg sodium | 8g carbohydrate | 2g fiber | 6g sugar | 2g protein | 30mg calcium | 300mg potassium | 40mg phosphorus | 1mg iron | 0mcg vitamin D

Grilled Radicchio Quarters

Prep Time: 5 minutes | **Cooking Time:** 6 minutes | **Total Time:** 11 minutes | **Serving:** 4 | **Difficulty:** Easy

Ingredients:

- 2 heads radicchio, quartered lengthwise
- 2 tablespoons olive oil
- Salt and pepper, to taste
- Balsamic vinegar (optional, for those who can tolerate it)

Instructions:

1. Preheat your grill to medium-high heat.

2. Brush the radicchio quarters with olive oil and season with salt and pepper.

3. Place the radicchio quarters on the grill and cook for 2-3 minutes on each side, or until slightly charred and wilted.

4. Drizzle with balsamic vinegar if desired.

5. Serve warm.

Nutritional Value:
60 calories | 5g fat | 1g saturated fat | 0mg cholesterol | 40mg sodium | 4g carbohydrate | 1g fiber | 2g sugar | 1g protein | 20mg calcium | 150mg potassium | 30mg phosphorus | 0.5mg iron | 0mcg vitamin D

Steamed Romanesco

Prep Time: 5 minutes | **Cooking Time:** 10 minutes | **Total Time:** 15 minutes | **Serving:** 4 | **Difficulty:** Easy

Ingredients:

- 1 head Romanesco, cut into florets
- 2 tablespoons olive oil
- Salt and pepper, to taste
- Fresh parsley, chopped (optional for garnish)

Instructions:

1. In a large pot, bring about 1 inch of water to a boil. Place a steamer basket in the pot.

2. Add the Romanesco florets to the steamer basket.

3. Cover and steam the Romanesco for 8-10 minutes, or until tender.

4. Transfer the steamed Romanesco to a serving bowl and drizzle with olive oil.

5. Season with salt and pepper to taste, and garnish with fresh parsley if desired.

6. Serve warm.

Nutritional Value:
80 calories | 7g fat | 1g saturated fat | 0mg cholesterol | 50mg sodium | 4g carbohydrate | 2g fiber | 2g sugar | 2g protein | 30mg calcium | 270mg potassium | 40mg phosphorus | 1mg iron | 0mcg vitamin D

Grilled Belgian Endive

Prep Time: 5 minutes | **Cooking Time:** 6 minutes | **Total Time:** 11 minutes | **Serving:** 4 | **Difficulty:** Easy

Ingredients:

- 4 heads Belgian endive, halved lengthwise

- 2 tablespoons olive oil

- Salt and pepper, to taste

Instructions:

1. Preheat your grill to medium-high heat.

2. Brush the cut sides of the Belgian endive with olive oil and season with salt and pepper.

3. Place the endive on the grill, cut side down, and cook for 3-4 minutes until lightly charred and tender.

4. Serve warm.

Nutritional Value:
60 calories | 5g fat | 1g saturated fat | 0mg cholesterol | 20mg sodium | 4g carbohydrate | 2g fiber | 1g sugar | 1g protein | 40mg calcium | 200mg potassium | 40mg phosphorus | 0.5mg iron | 0mcg vitamin D

Steamed Mustard Greens

Prep Time: 5 minutes | **Cooking Time:** 8 minutes | **Total Time:** 13 minutes | **Serving:** 4 | **Difficulty:** Easy

Ingredients:

- 8 cups mustard greens, washed and chopped

- 2 tablespoons olive oil

- 2 cloves garlic, minced

- Salt and pepper, to taste

Instructions:

1. In a large pot, bring about 1 inch of water to a boil. Place a steamer basket in the pot.

2. Add the chopped mustard greens to the steamer basket.

3. Cover and steam the mustard greens for 6-8 minutes, or until wilted and tender.

4. In a small saucepan, heat the olive oil over medium heat. Add the minced garlic and sauté until fragrant, about 1 minute.

5. Drizzle the garlic oil over the steamed mustard greens.

6. Season with salt and pepper to taste.

7. Serve hot.

Nutritional Value:

80 calories | 5g fat | 1g saturated fat | 0mg cholesterol | 60mg sodium | 7g carbohydrate | 4g fiber | 1g sugar | 3g protein | 80mg calcium | 600mg potassium | 40mg phosphorus | 2mg iron | 0mcg vitamin D

Steamed Collard Greens

Prep Time: 5 minutes | **Cooking Time:** 8 minutes | **Total Time:** 13 minutes | **Serving:** 4 | **Difficulty:** Easy

Ingredients:

- 8 cups collard greens, washed and chopped
- 2 tablespoons olive oil
- 2 cloves garlic, minced
- Salt and pepper, to taste

Instructions:

1. In a large pot, bring about 1 inch of water to a boil. Place a steamer basket in the pot.

2. Add the chopped collard greens to the steamer basket.

3. Cover and steam the collard greens for 6-8 minutes, or until wilted and tender.

4. In a small saucepan, heat the olive oil over medium heat. Add the minced garlic and sauté until fragrant, about 1 minute.

5. Drizzle the garlic oil over the steamed collard greens.

6. Season with salt and pepper to taste.

7. Serve hot.

Nutritional Value:

80 calories | 5g fat | 1g saturated fat | 0mg cholesterol | 60mg sodium | 7g carbohydrate | 4g fiber | 1g sugar | 3g protein | 80mg calcium | 600mg potassium | 40mg phosphorus | 2mg iron | 0mcg vitamin D

Steamed Haricot Verts

Prep Time: 5 minutes | **Cooking Time:** 6 minutes | **Total Time:** 11 minutes | **Serving:** 4 | **Difficulty:** Easy

Ingredients:

- 4 cups haricot verts (French green beans), trimmed
- 2 tablespoons olive oil
- Salt and pepper, to taste
- Fresh lemon zest (optional)

Instructions:

1. In a large pot, bring about 1 inch of water to a boil. Place a steamer basket in the pot.

2. Add the haricot verts to the steamer basket.

3. Cover and steam the haricot verts for 5-6 minutes, or until tender-crisp.

4. Transfer the steamed haricot verts to a serving bowl and drizzle with olive oil.

5. Season with salt and pepper to taste, and garnish with fresh lemon zest if desired.

6. Serve hot.

Nutritional Value:

70 calories | 5g fat | 1g saturated fat | 0mg cholesterol | 20mg sodium | 5g carbohydrate | 2g fiber | 2g sugar | 2g protein | 20mg calcium | 180mg potassium | 40mg phosphorus | 1mg iron | 0mcg vitamin D

Steamed Turnip Greens

Prep Time: 5 minutes | **Cooking Time:** 8 minutes | **Total Time:** 13 minutes | **Serving:** 4 | **Difficulty:** Easy

Ingredients:

- 8 cups turnip greens, washed and chopped
- 2 tablespoons olive oil
- 2 cloves garlic, minced
- Salt and pepper, to taste

Instructions:

1. In a large pot, bring about 1 inch of water to a boil. Place a steamer basket in the pot.

2. Add the chopped turnip greens to the steamer basket.

3. Cover and steam the turnip greens for 6-8 minutes, or until wilted and tender.

4. In a small saucepan, heat the olive oil over medium heat. Add the minced garlic and sauté until fragrant, about 1 minute.

5. Drizzle the garlic oil over the steamed turnip greens.

6. Season with salt and pepper to taste.

7. Serve hot.

Nutritional Value:

80 calories | 5g fat | 1g saturated fat | 0mg cholesterol | 60mg sodium | 7g carbohydrate | 4g fiber | 1g sugar | 3g protein | 80mg calcium | 600mg potassium | 40mg phosphorus | 2mg iron | 0mcg vitamin D

Steamed Dandelion Greens

Prep Time: 5 minutes | **Cooking Time:** 8 minutes | **Total Time:** 13 minutes | **Serving:** 4 | **Difficulty:** Easy

Ingredients:

- 8 cups dandelion greens, washed and trimmed

- 2 tablespoons olive oil

- 2 cloves garlic, minced

- Salt and pepper, to taste

Instructions:

1. In a large pot, bring about 1 inch of water to a boil. Place a steamer basket in the pot.

2. Add the dandelion greens to the steamer basket.

3. Cover and steam the dandelion greens for 6-8 minutes, or until wilted and tender.

4. In a small saucepan, heat the olive oil over medium heat. Add the

minced garlic and sauté until fragrant, about 1 minute.

5. Drizzle the garlic oil over the steamed dandelion greens.

6. Season with salt and pepper to taste.

7. Serve hot.

Nutritional Value:

80 calories | 5g fat | 1g saturated fat | 0mg cholesterol | 60mg sodium | 7g carbohydrate | 4g fiber | 1g sugar | 3g protein | 80mg calcium | 600mg potassium | 40mg phosphorus | 2mg iron | 0mcg vitamin D

Steamed Rapini

Prep Time: 5 minutes | **Cooking Time:** 6 minutes | **Total Time:** 11 minutes | **Serving:** 4 | **Difficulty:** Easy

Ingredients:

- 8 cups rapini (broccoli rabe), washed and trimmed

- 2 tablespoons olive oil

- 2 cloves garlic, minced

- Salt and pepper, to taste

Instructions:

1. In a large pot, bring about 1 inch of water to a boil. Place a steamer basket in the pot.

2. Add the rapini to the steamer basket.

3. Cover and steam the rapini for 5-6 minutes, or until tender.

4. In a small saucepan, heat the olive oil over medium heat. Add the minced garlic and sauté until fragrant, about 1 minute.

5. Drizzle the garlic oil over the steamed rapini.

6. Season with salt and pepper to taste.

7. Serve hot.

Nutritional Value:
70 calories | 5g fat | 1g saturated fat | 0mg cholesterol | 60mg sodium | 5g carbohydrate | 2g fiber | 1g sugar | 2g protein | 80mg calcium | 500mg potassium | 40mg phosphorus | 2mg iron | 0mcg vitamin D

Steamed Watercress

Prep Time: 5 minutes | **Cooking Time:** 5 minutes | **Total Time:** 10 minutes | **Serving:** 4 | **Difficulty:** Easy

Ingredients:

- 4 cups fresh watercress, washed and trimmed

- 2 tablespoons olive oil

- 1 clove garlic, minced

- Salt and pepper, to taste

Instructions:

1. In a large pot, bring about 1 inch of water to a boil. Place a steamer basket in the pot.

2. Add the watercress to the steamer basket.

3. Cover and steam the watercress for 3-5 minutes, or until wilted and tender.

4. In a small saucepan, heat the olive oil over medium heat. Add the minced garlic and sauté until fragrant, about 1 minute.

5. Drizzle the garlic oil over the steamed watercress.

6. Season with salt and pepper to taste.

7. Serve hot.

Nutritional Value:
60 calories | 5g fat | 0.5g saturated fat | 0mg cholesterol | 40mg sodium | 3g carbohydrate | 1g fiber | 0g sugar | 2g protein | 40mg calcium | 220mg potassium | 40mg phosphorus | 1mg iron | 0mcg vitamin D

Steamed Fiddlehead Ferns

Prep Time: 5 minutes | **Cooking Time:** 10 minutes | **Total Time:** 15 minutes | **Serving:** 4 | **Difficulty:** Easy

Ingredients:

- 4 cups fresh fiddlehead ferns, cleaned and trimmed
- 2 tablespoons olive oil
- 1 tablespoon lemon juice (optional, for those who can tolerate it)
- Salt and pepper, to taste

Instructions:

1. In a large pot, bring about 1 inch of water to a boil. Place a steamer basket in the pot.
2. Add the fiddlehead ferns to the steamer basket.
3. Cover and steam the fiddleheads for 8-10 minutes, or until tender.
4. Transfer the steamed fiddlehead ferns to a serving bowl and drizzle with olive oil.
5. If using, add a squeeze of lemon juice.
6. Season with salt and pepper to taste.
7. Serve hot.

Nutritional Value:

70 calories | 5g fat | 0.5g saturated fat | 0mg cholesterol | 40mg sodium | 6g carbohydrate | 2g fiber | 0g sugar | 3g protein | 50mg calcium | 300mg potassium | 40mg phosphorus | 2mg iron | 0mcg vitamin D

Steamed Sea Beans

Prep Time: 5 minutes | **Cooking Time:** 5 minutes | **Total Time:** 10 minutes | **Serving:** 4 | **Difficulty:** Easy

Ingredients:

- 4 cups sea beans, cleaned and trimmed
- 2 tablespoons olive oil
- 1 clove garlic, minced
- Salt and pepper, to taste

Instructions:

1. In a large pot, bring about 1 inch of water to a boil. Place a steamer basket in the pot.
2. Add the sea beans to the steamer basket.
3. Cover and steam the sea beans for 3-5 minutes, or until tender.
4. In a small saucepan, heat the olive oil over medium heat. Add the minced garlic and sauté until fragrant, about 1 minute.
5. Drizzle the garlic oil over the steamed sea beans.

6. Season with salt and pepper to taste.

7. Serve hot.

Nutritional Value:
60 calories | 5g fat | 0.5g saturated fat | 0mg cholesterol | 40mg sodium | 4g carbohydrate | 2g fiber | 0g sugar | 2g protein | 30mg calcium | 300mg potassium | 40mg phosphorus | 1mg iron | 0mcg vitamin D

Steamed Pea Shoots

Prep Time: 5 minutes | **Cooking Time:** 5 minutes | **Total Time:** 10 minutes | **Serving:** 4 | **Difficulty:** Easy

Ingredients:

- 4 cups fresh pea shoots, washed and trimmed

- 2 tablespoons olive oil

- 1 clove garlic, minced

- Salt and pepper, to taste

Instructions:

1. In a large pot, bring about 1 inch of water to a boil. Place a steamer basket in the pot.

2. Add the pea shoots to the steamer basket.

3. Cover and steam the pea shoots for 3-5 minutes, or until wilted and tender.

4. In a small saucepan, heat the olive oil over medium heat. Add the minced garlic and sauté until fragrant, about 1 minute.

5. Drizzle the garlic oil over the steamed pea shoots.

6. Season with salt and pepper to taste.

7. Serve hot.

Nutritional Value:
60 calories | 5g fat | 0.5g saturated fat | 0mg cholesterol | 40mg sodium | 3g carbohydrate | 1g fiber | 1g sugar | 2g protein | 40mg calcium | 200mg potassium | 40mg phosphorus | 1mg iron | 0mcg vitamin D

Dear Reader,

Thank you for choosing "**Ulcer Diet Cookbook for Beginners: Simple, Nourishing Recipes to Support Your Gut and manage Symptoms.**" I truly hope this book provides you with the comfort, guidance, and practical meal solutions you need to support your healing journey.

If this book has been helpful to you, I would greatly appreciate it if you could take a moment to leave an honest review on Amazon. Your feedback not only helps other facing similar challenges but also allows me to continue creating resources that make a difference in families' lives.

Whether it's sharing what you found most useful or offering suggestions for improvement, your review matters and will help others make informed decisions.

Thank you so much for your support and for being part of this journey toward better health.

Warmly,

Elena Richard

Grains and Starches

Vegetable Risotto

Prep Time: 15 minutes | **Cooking Time:** 30 minutes | **Total Time:** 45 minutes | **Serving:** 4 | **Difficulty:** Easy

Ingredients:

- 1 cup Arborio rice
- 4 cups low-sodium vegetable broth
- 1 small onion, finely chopped
- 1 garlic clove, minced
- 1 cup diced zucchini
- 1 cup diced carrots
- 1/2 cup frozen peas
- 2 tablespoons olive oil
- 1/4 cup grated Parmesan cheese (optional)
- Salt and pepper, to taste
- Fresh parsley, chopped (optional for garnish)

Instructions:

1. In a large saucepan, heat the olive oil over medium heat. Add the chopped onion and garlic, sautéing until softened, about 3 minutes.

2. Add the Arborio rice and cook, stirring constantly, for 2-3 minutes until the rice is lightly toasted.

3. Begin adding the vegetable broth, one cup at a time, stirring frequently. Wait until the broth is almost fully absorbed before adding the next cup. Continue this process until the rice is creamy and cooked through, about 18-20 minutes.

4. Stir in the zucchini, carrots, and peas, and cook for an additional 5-7 minutes until the vegetables are tender.

5. If using, stir in the Parmesan cheese and season with salt and pepper to taste.

6. Serve hot, garnished with fresh parsley if desired.

Nutritional Value:

350 calories | 9g fat | 2g saturated fat | 5mg cholesterol | 220mg sodium | 54g carbohydrate | 4g fiber | 4g sugar | 9g protein | 80mg calcium | 300mg potassium | 100mg phosphorus | 1mg iron | 0mcg vitamin D

Baked Sweet Potato

Prep Time: 5 minutes | **Cooking Time:** 45 minutes | **Total Time:** 50 minutes | **Serving:** 4 | **Difficulty:** Easy

Ingredients:

- 4 medium sweet potatoes, washed
- 2 tablespoons olive oil
- Salt and pepper, to taste
- Ground cinnamon (optional)

Instructions:

1. Preheat your oven to 400°F (200°C).

2. Place the sweet potatoes on a baking sheet. Using a fork, pierce each potato several times.

3. Drizzle the sweet potatoes with olive oil and rub to coat evenly.

4. Bake for 45-50 minutes, or until the sweet potatoes are tender when pierced with a fork.

5. Remove from the oven and let cool slightly before slicing open.

6. Season with salt, pepper, and a sprinkle of ground cinnamon if desired.

7. Serve hot.

Nutritional Value:

180 calories | 7g fat | 1g saturated fat | 0mg cholesterol | 40mg sodium | 29g carbohydrate | 5g fiber | 9g sugar | 2g protein | 40mg calcium | 440mg potassium | 80mg phosphorus | 1mg iron | 0mcg vitamin D

Vegetable Quinoa Pilaf

Prep Time: 10 minutes | **Cooking Time:** 20 minutes | **Total Time:** 30 minutes | **Serving:** 4 | **Difficulty:** Easy

Ingredients:

- 1 cup quinoa, rinsed
- 2 cups low-sodium vegetable broth
- 1 small onion, finely chopped
- 1 garlic clove, minced
- 1 cup diced bell peppers (red, yellow, or green)
- 1 cup diced zucchini
- 1/2 cup grated carrots
- 2 tablespoons olive oil
- Salt and pepper, to taste
- Fresh parsley, chopped (optional for garnish)

Instructions:

1. In a medium saucepan, heat the olive oil over medium heat. Add the chopped onion and garlic, sautéing until softened, about 3 minutes.

2. Add the rinsed quinoa and cook, stirring constantly, for 2 minutes.

3. Pour in the vegetable broth and bring to a boil. Reduce the heat to low, cover, and simmer for 15

minutes, or until the quinoa is cooked and the liquid is absorbed.

4. While the quinoa is cooking, in a separate skillet, sauté the diced bell peppers, zucchini, and grated carrots until tender, about 5 minutes.

5. Fluff the cooked quinoa with a fork and stir in the sautéed vegetables. Season with salt and pepper to taste.

6. Serve hot, garnished with fresh parsley if desired.

Nutritional Value:
220 calories | 8g fat | 1g saturated fat | 0mg cholesterol | 180mg sodium | 32g carbohydrate | 5g fiber | 3g sugar | 7g protein | 40mg calcium | 400mg potassium | 150mg phosphorus | 2mg iron | 0mcg vitamin D

Vegetable Couscous

Prep Time: 10 minutes | **Cooking Time:** 10 minutes | **Total Time:** 20 minutes | **Serving:** 4 | **Difficulty:** Easy

Ingredients:

- 1 cup whole wheat couscous
- 1 cup low-sodium vegetable broth
- 1 small zucchini, diced
- 1 small carrot, grated
- 1/2 cup frozen peas
- 2 tablespoons olive oil

- 1 garlic clove, minced
- Salt and pepper, to taste
- Fresh mint, chopped (optional for garnish)

Instructions:

1. In a medium saucepan, bring the vegetable broth to a boil. Remove from heat, add the couscous, cover, and let sit for 5 minutes.

2. Meanwhile, in a skillet, heat the olive oil over medium heat. Add the garlic and sauté until fragrant, about 1 minute.

3. Add the diced zucchini, grated carrot, and peas to the skillet, and sauté for 5 minutes until the vegetables are tender.

4. Fluff the couscous with a fork and stir in the sautéed vegetables. Season with salt and pepper to taste.

5. Serve hot, garnished with fresh mint if desired.

Nutritional Value:
200 calories | 7g fat | 1g saturated fat | 0mg cholesterol | 150mg sodium | 31g carbohydrate | 5g fiber | 3g sugar | 5g protein | 20mg calcium | 300mg potassium | 80mg phosphorus | 1mg iron | 0mcg vitamin D

Baked Sweet Potato Fries

Prep Time: 10 minutes | **Cooking Time:** 30 minutes | **Total Time:** 40 minutes | **Serving:** 4 | **Difficulty:** Easy

Ingredients:

- 4 medium sweet potatoes, peeled and cut into 1/4-inch thick fries
- 2 tablespoons olive oil
- 1 teaspoon garlic powder
- 1/2 teaspoon paprika
- Salt and pepper, to taste

Instructions:

1. Preheat your oven to 425°F (220°C).
2. In a large bowl, toss the sweet potato fries with olive oil, garlic powder, paprika, salt, and pepper.
3. Spread the fries in a single layer on a baking sheet lined with parchment paper.
4. Bake for 25-30 minutes, flipping halfway through, until the fries are crispy and golden brown.
5. Serve hot.

Nutritional Value:

180 calories | 7g fat | 1g saturated fat | 0mg cholesterol | 160mg sodium | 27g carbohydrate | 5g fiber | 6g sugar | 2g protein | 40mg calcium | 400mg potassium | 80mg phosphorus | 1mg iron | 0mcg vitamin

D

Baked Spaghetti Squash

Prep Time: 10 minutes | **Cooking Time:** 40 minutes | **Total Time:** 50 minutes | **Serving:** 4 | **Difficulty:** Easy

Ingredients:

- 1 medium spaghetti squash
- 2 tablespoons olive oil
- Salt and pepper, to taste
- Fresh basil, chopped (optional for garnish)

Instructions:

1. Preheat your oven to 400°F (200°C).
2. Cut the spaghetti squash in half lengthwise and scoop out the seeds.
3. Drizzle the inside of each half with olive oil and season with salt and pepper.
4. Place the squash halves cut side down on a baking sheet lined with parchment paper.
5. Bake for 40 minutes, or until the squash is tender and easily pierced with a fork.
6. Remove from the oven and let cool slightly. Use a fork to scrape out the strands of squash.

7. Serve hot, garnished with fresh basil if desired.

Nutritional Value:
110 calories | 7g fat | 1g saturated fat | 0mg cholesterol | 80mg sodium | 12g carbohydrate | 3g fiber | 4g sugar | 1g protein | 40mg calcium | 180mg potassium | 60mg phosphorus | 0.5mg iron | 0mcg vitamin D

Baked Turnip Fries

Prep Time: 10 minutes | **Cooking Time:** 30 minutes | **Total Time:** 40 minutes | **Serving:** 4 | **Difficulty:** Easy

Ingredients:

- 4 medium turnips, peeled and cut into 1/4-inch thick fries

- 2 tablespoons olive oil

- 1 teaspoon garlic powder

- 1/2 teaspoon paprika

- Salt and pepper, to taste

Instructions:

1. Preheat your oven to 425°F (220°C).

2. In a large bowl, toss the turnip fries with olive oil, garlic powder, paprika, salt, and pepper.

3. Spread the fries in a single layer on a baking sheet lined with parchment paper.

4. Bake for 25-30 minutes, flipping halfway through, until the fries are crispy and golden brown.

5. Serve hot.

Nutritional Value:
120 calories | 7g fat | 1g saturated fat | 0mg cholesterol | 160mg sodium | 14g carbohydrate | 3g fiber | 4g sugar | 2g protein | 40mg calcium | 300mg potassium | 60mg phosphorus | 0.5mg iron | 0mcg vitamin D

Baked Rutabaga Wedges

Prep Time: 10 minutes | **Cooking Time:** 40 minutes | **Total Time:** 50 minutes | **Serving:** 4 | **Difficulty:** Easy

Ingredients:

- 2 medium rutabagas, peeled and cut into wedges

- 2 tablespoons olive oil

- 1 teaspoon dried thyme

- Salt and pepper, to taste

Instructions:

1. Preheat your oven to 400°F (200°C).

2. In a large bowl, toss the rutabaga wedges with olive oil, thyme, salt, and pepper.

3. Spread the wedges in a single layer on a baking sheet lined with parchment paper.

4. Bake for 35-40 minutes, flipping halfway through, until the wedges are golden brown and tender.

5. Serve hot.

Nutritional Value:

140 calories | 7g fat | 1g saturated fat | 0mg cholesterol | 160mg sodium | 18g carbohydrate | 5g fiber | 7g sugar | 2g protein | 60mg calcium | 500mg potassium | 80mg phosphorus | 1mg iron | 0mcg vitamin D

Baked Kohlrabi Fries

Prep Time: 10 minutes | **Cooking Time:** 30 minutes | **Total Time:** 40 minutes | **Serving:** 4 | **Difficulty:** Easy

Ingredients:

- 4 medium kohlrabi, peeled and cut into 1/4-inch thick fries

- 2 tablespoons olive oil

- 1 teaspoon garlic powder

- 1/2 teaspoon smoked paprika

- Salt and pepper, to taste

Instructions:

1. Preheat your oven to 425°F (220°C).

2. In a large bowl, toss the kohlrabi fries with olive oil, garlic powder, smoked paprika, salt, and pepper.

3. Spread the fries in a single layer on a baking sheet lined with parchment paper.

4. Bake for 25-30 minutes, flipping halfway through, until the fries are crispy and golden brown.

5. Serve hot.

Nutritional Value:

130 calories | 7g fat | 1g saturated fat | 0mg cholesterol | 160mg sodium | 12g carbohydrate | 4g fiber | 6g sugar | 3g protein | 60mg calcium | 400mg potassium | 80mg phosphorus | 1mg iron | 0mcg vitamin D

Baked Delicata Squash Rings

Prep Time: 10 minutes | **Cooking Time:** 20 minutes | **Total Time:** 30 minutes | **Serving:** 4 | **Difficulty:** Easy

Ingredients:

- 2 medium delicata squashes, halved, seeds removed, and sliced into rings

- 2 tablespoons olive oil

- 1 teaspoon dried thyme

- 1/2 teaspoon ground cinnamon (optional)

- Salt and pepper, to taste

Instructions:

1. Preheat your oven to 400°F (200°C).

2. In a large bowl, toss the delicata squash rings with olive oil, thyme, cinnamon (if using), salt, and pepper.

3. Arrange the rings in a single layer on a baking sheet lined with parchment paper.

4. Bake for 20-25 minutes, flipping halfway through, until the rings are tender and golden brown.

5. Serve hot.

Nutritional Value:
110 calories | 7g fat | 1g saturated fat | 0mg cholesterol | 60mg sodium | 14g carbohydrate | 3g fiber | 4g sugar | 1g protein | 40mg calcium | 200mg potassium | 40mg phosphorus | 0.5mg iron | 0mcg vitamin D

Baked Yam Wedges

Prep Time: 10 minutes | **Cooking Time:** 30 minutes | **Total Time:** 40 minutes | **Serving:** 4 | **Difficulty:** Easy

Ingredients:

- 2 large yams, peeled and cut into wedges

- 2 tablespoons olive oil

- 1 teaspoon garlic powder

- 1 teaspoon paprika

- Salt and pepper, to taste

Instructions:

1. Preheat your oven to 400°F (200°C).

2. In a large bowl, toss the yam wedges with olive oil, garlic powder, paprika, salt, and pepper.

3. Spread the wedges in a single layer on a baking sheet lined with parchment paper.

4. Bake for 25-30 minutes, flipping halfway through, until the wedges are golden brown and tender.

5. Serve hot.

Nutritional Value:
160 calories | 7g fat | 1g saturated fat | 0mg cholesterol | 160mg sodium | 23g carbohydrate | 4g fiber | 6g sugar | 2g protein | 50mg calcium | 450mg potassium | 90mg phosphorus | 1mg iron | 0mcg vitamin D

Baked Jicama Fries

Prep Time: 10 minutes | **Cooking Time:** 40 minutes | **Total Time:** 50 minutes | **Serving:** 4 | **Difficulty:** Easy

Ingredients:

- 1 large jicama, peeled and cut into fries

- 2 tablespoons olive oil

- 1 teaspoon garlic powder

- 1/2 teaspoon paprika

- Salt and pepper, to taste

Instructions:

1. Preheat your oven to 400°F (200°C).

2. In a large bowl, toss the jicama fries with olive oil, garlic powder, paprika, salt, and pepper.

3. Spread the fries in a single layer on a baking sheet lined with parchment paper.

4. Bake for 35-40 minutes, flipping halfway through, until the fries are crispy and golden brown.

5. Serve hot.

Nutritional Value:

110 calories | 6g fat | 1g saturated fat | 0mg cholesterol | 160mg sodium | 15g carbohydrate | 7g fiber | 3g sugar | 1g protein | 30mg calcium | 250mg potassium | 60mg phosphorus | 0.5mg iron | 0mcg vitamin D

Baked Carrot Chips

Prep Time: 10 minutes | **Cooking Time:** 20 minutes | **Total Time:** 30 minutes | **Serving:** 4 | **Difficulty:** Easy

Ingredients:

- 4 large carrots, peeled and sliced thinly into rounds

- 2 tablespoons olive oil

- 1 teaspoon ground cumin

- Salt and pepper, to taste

Instructions:

1. Preheat your oven to 400°F (200°C).

2. In a large bowl, toss the carrot slices with olive oil, ground cumin, salt, and pepper.

3. Spread the slices in a single layer on a baking sheet lined with parchment paper.

4. Bake for 15-20 minutes, flipping halfway through, until the chips are crispy and lightly browned.

5. Serve hot.

Nutritional Value:

80 calories | 5g fat | 1g saturated fat | 0mg cholesterol | 150mg sodium | 9g carbohydrate | 3g fiber | 4g sugar | 1g protein | 30mg calcium | 300mg potassium | 40mg phosphorus | 0.5mg iron | 0mcg vitamin D

Baked Cassava Wedges

Prep Time: 10 minutes | **Cooking Time:** 30 minutes | **Total Time:** 40 minutes | **Serving:** 4 | **Difficulty:** Easy

Ingredients:

- 2 large cassava roots, peeled and cut into wedges

- 2 tablespoons olive oil

- 1 teaspoon garlic powder

- 1 teaspoon smoked paprika

- Salt and pepper, to taste

Instructions:

1. Preheat your oven to 400°F (200°C).

2. In a large bowl, toss the cassava wedges with olive oil, garlic powder, smoked paprika, salt, and pepper.

3. Spread the wedges in a single layer on a baking sheet lined with parchment paper.

4. Bake for 25-30 minutes, flipping halfway through, until the wedges are golden brown and crispy.

5. Serve hot.

Nutritional Value:

200 calories | 8g fat | 1g saturated fat | 0mg cholesterol | 160mg sodium | 30g carbohydrate | 3g fiber | 2g sugar | 2g protein | 40mg calcium | 300mg potassium | 90mg phosphorus | 1mg iron | 0mcg vitamin D

Baked Taro Chips

Prep Time: 10 minutes | **Cooking Time:** 20 minutes | **Total Time:** 30 minutes | **Serving:** 4 | **Difficulty:** Easy

Ingredients:

- 2 large taro roots, peeled and thinly sliced into rounds

- 2 tablespoons olive oil

- 1 teaspoon ground turmeric

- Salt and pepper, to taste

Instructions:

1. Preheat your oven to 375°F (190°C).

2. In a large bowl, toss the taro slices with olive oil, ground turmeric, salt, and pepper.

3. Spread the slices in a single layer on a baking sheet lined with parchment paper.

4. Bake for 15-20 minutes, flipping halfway through, until the chips are crispy and lightly browned.

5. Serve hot.

Nutritional Value:

140 calories | 7g fat | 1g saturated fat | 0mg cholesterol | 160mg sodium | 18g carbohydrate | 3g fiber | 1g sugar | 2g protein | 20mg calcium | 200mg potassium | 50mg phosphorus | 0.5mg iron | 0mcg vitamin D

Baked Lotus Root Chips

Prep Time: 10 minutes | **Cooking Time:** 20 minutes | **Total Time:** 30 minutes | **Serving:** 4 | **Difficulty:** Easy

Ingredients:

- 2 medium lotus roots, peeled and thinly sliced into rounds
- 2 tablespoons olive oil
- 1 teaspoon garlic powder
- Salt and pepper, to taste

Instructions:

1. Preheat your oven to 375°F (190°C).
2. In a large bowl, toss the lotus root slices with olive oil, garlic powder, salt, and pepper.
3. Spread the slices in a single layer on a baking sheet lined with parchment paper.
4. Bake for 15 20 minutes, flipping halfway through, until the chips are crispy and lightly browned.
5. Serve hot.

Nutritional Value:
120 calories | 6g fat | 1g saturated fat | 0mg cholesterol | 160mg sodium | 18g carbohydrate | 4g fiber | 2g sugar | 2g protein | 20mg calcium | 200mg potassium | 50mg phosphorus | 0.5mg iron | 0mcg vitamin D

Baked Kabocha Squash Wedges

Prep Time: 10 minutes | **Cooking Time:** 30 minutes | **Total Time:** 40 minutes | **Serving:** 4 | **Difficulty:** Easy

Ingredients:

- 1 medium kabocha squash, seeded and cut into wedges
- 2 tablespoons olive oil
- 1 teaspoon ground cinnamon
- 1/4 teaspoon ground nutmeg (optional)
- Salt and pepper, to taste

Instructions:

1. Preheat your oven to 400°F (200°C).
2. In a large bowl, toss the kabocha squash wedges with olive oil, cinnamon, nutmeg (if using), salt, and pepper.
3. Spread the wedges in a single layer on a baking sheet lined with parchment paper.
4. Bake for 25-30 minutes, flipping halfway through, until the wedges are tender and golden brown.
5. Serve hot.

Nutritional Value:
140 calories | 7g fat | 1g saturated fat | 0mg cholesterol | 160mg sodium | 18g carbohydrate | 4g fiber | 6g sugar | 2g

protein | 60mg calcium | 400mg potassium | 80mg phosphorus | 1mg iron | 0mcg vitamin D

protein | 40mg calcium | 300mg potassium | 60mg phosphorus | 1mg iron | 0mcg vitamin D

Baked Okra Chips

Prep Time: 10 minutes | **Cooking Time:** 25 minutes | **Total Time:** 35 minutes | **Serving:** 4 | **Difficulty:** Easy

Ingredients:

- 4 cups okra, trimmed and halved lengthwise
- 2 tablespoons olive oil
- 1 teaspoon smoked paprika
- Salt and pepper, to taste

Instructions:

1. Preheat your oven to 400°F (200°C).
2. In a large bowl, toss the okra halves with olive oil, smoked paprika, salt, and pepper.
3. Spread the okra in a single layer on a baking sheet lined with parchment paper.
4. Bake for 20-25 minutes, flipping halfway through, until the okra is crispy and lightly browned.
5. Serve hot.

Nutritional Value:

100 calories | 6g fat | 1g saturated fat | 0mg cholesterol | 160mg sodium | 12g carbohydrate | 5g fiber | 2g sugar | 2g

Baked Chayote Squash

Prep Time: 10 minutes | **Cooking Time:** 30 minutes | **Total Time:** 40 minutes | **Serving:** 4 | **Difficulty:** Easy

Ingredients:

- 2 medium chayote squashes, peeled, cored, and sliced
- 2 tablespoons olive oil
- 1 teaspoon dried thyme
- Salt and pepper, to taste

Instructions:

1. Preheat your oven to 400°F (200°C).
2. In a large bowl, toss the chayote slices with olive oil, thyme, salt, and pepper.
3. Spread the slices in a single layer on a baking sheet lined with parchment paper.
4. Bake for 25-30 minutes, flipping halfway through, until the slices are tender and lightly browned.
5. Serve hot.

Nutritional Value:

80 calories | 5g fat | 1g saturated fat | 0mg cholesterol | 160mg sodium | 10g carbohydrate | 4g fiber | 2g sugar | 1g

protein | 20mg calcium | 200mg potassium | 40mg phosphorus | 0.5mg iron | 0mcg vitamin D

Baked Sunchoke Chips

Prep Time: 10 minutes | **Cooking Time:** 25 minutes | **Total Time:** 35 minutes | **Serving:** 4 | **Difficulty:** Easy

Ingredients:

- 4 medium sunchokes (Jerusalem artichokes), peeled and thinly sliced
- 2 tablespoons olive oil
- 1 teaspoon garlic powder
- Salt and pepper, to taste

Instructions:

1. Preheat your oven to 375°F (190°C).

2. In a large bowl, toss the sunchoke slices with olive oil, garlic powder, salt, and pepper.

3. Spread the slices in a single layer on a baking sheet lined with parchment paper.

4. Bake for 20-25 minutes, flipping halfway through, until the chips are crispy and lightly browned.

5. Serve hot.

Nutritional Value:

120 calories | 7g fat | 1g saturated fat | 0mg cholesterol | 160mg sodium | 16g carbohydrate | 3g fiber | 2g sugar | 2g protein | 20mg calcium | 200mg potassium | 50mg phosphorus | 0.5mg iron | 0mcg vitamin D

Fruit Dishes

Poached Pear Dessert

Prep Time: 10 minutes | **Cooking Time:** 20 minutes | **Total Time:** 30 minutes | **Serving:** 4 | **Difficulty:** Easy

Ingredients:

- 4 ripe pears, peeled and cored
- 4 cups water
- 1/2 cup honey or maple syrup
- 1 cinnamon stick
- 1 vanilla bean, split (or 1 teaspoon vanilla extract)
- 2-3 whole cloves (optional)

Instructions:

1. In a large saucepan, combine the water, honey or maple syrup, cinnamon stick, vanilla bean (or extract), and cloves (if using). Bring to a simmer over medium heat.
2. Add the pears to the saucepan, making sure they are fully submerged in the liquid.
3. Reduce the heat to low and poach the pears for 15-20 minutes, or until they are tender when pierced with a fork.
4. Remove the pears from the liquid and let them cool slightly before serving.
5. Serve warm or chilled, with a drizzle of the poaching liquid.

Nutritional Value:

180 calories | 0g fat | 0g saturated fat | 0mg cholesterol | 10mg sodium | 45g carbohydrate | 5g fiber | 30g sugar | 1g protein | 20mg calcium | 200mg potassium | 40mg phosphorus | 0.5mg iron | 0mcg vitamin D

Grilled Peaches with Yogurt

Prep Time: 5 minutes | **Cooking Time:** 6 minutes | **Total Time:** 11 minutes | **Serving:** 4 | **Difficulty:** Easy

Ingredients:

- 4 ripe peaches, halved and pitted
- 2 tablespoons honey or maple syrup
- 1 teaspoon ground cinnamon
- 1 cup plain Greek yogurt (optional)
- Fresh mint leaves for garnish (optional)

Instructions:

1. Preheat your grill to medium heat.

2. In a small bowl, mix together the honey or maple syrup and ground cinnamon.

3. Brush the cut sides of the peaches with the honey mixture.

4. Place the peaches cut side down on the grill and cook for 3-4 minutes, until grill marks appear and the peaches are slightly softened.

5. Remove the peaches from the grill and let cool slightly.

6. Serve the grilled peaches warm, topped with a dollop of Greek yogurt and a garnish of fresh mint if desired.

Nutritional Value:
120 calories | 2g fat | 1g saturated fat | 5mg cholesterol | 15mg sodium | 24g carbohydrate | 3g fiber | 20g sugar | 3g protein | 50mg calcium | 300mg potassium | 40mg phosphorus | 0.5mg iron | 0mcg vitamin D

Grilled Pineapple Slices

Prep Time: 5 minutes | **Cooking Time:** 6 minutes | **Total Time:** 11 minutes | **Serving:** 4 | **Difficulty:** Easy

Ingredients:

- 1 fresh pineapple, peeled, cored, and cut into 1/2-inch thick slices

- 2 tablespoons honey or maple syrup

- 1 teaspoon ground cinnamon

Instructions:

1. Preheat your grill to medium-high heat.

2. In a small bowl, mix together the honey or maple syrup and ground cinnamon.

3. Brush the pineapple slices with the honey mixture.

4. Place the pineapple slices on the grill and cook for 2-3 minutes on each side, until grill marks appear and the pineapple is caramelized.

5. Serve warm.

Nutritional Value:
100 calories | 0g fat | 0g saturated fat | 0mg cholesterol | 5mg sodium | 26g carbohydrate | 2g fiber | 22g sugar | 1g protein | 20mg calcium | 200mg potassium | 40mg phosphorus | 0.5mg iron | 0mcg vitamin D

Grilled Nectarine Halves

Prep Time: 5 minutes | **Cooking Time:** 6 minutes | **Total Time:** 11 minutes | **Serving:** 4 | **Difficulty:** Easy

Ingredients:

- 4 ripe nectarines, halved and pitted

- 2 tablespoons honey or maple syrup

- 1 teaspoon ground cinnamon

Instructions:

1. Preheat your grill to medium heat.

2. In a small bowl, mix together the honey or maple syrup and ground cinnamon.

3. Brush the cut sides of the nectarines with the honey mixture.

4. Place the nectarines cut side down on the grill and cook for 3-4 minutes, until grill marks appear and the nectarines are slightly softened.

5. Serve warm.

Nutritional Value:

90 calories | 0g fat | 0g saturated fat | 0mg cholesterol | 5mg sodium | 24g carbohydrate | 3g fiber | 20g sugar | 1g protein | 20mg calcium | 200mg potassium | 40mg phosphorus | 0.5mg iron | 0mcg vitamin D

Baked Apple Chips

Prep Time: 10 minutes | **Cooking Time:** 2 hours | **Total Time:** 2 hours 10 minutes | **Serving:** 4 | **Difficulty:** Easy

Ingredients:

- 4 large apples, cored and thinly sliced into rounds

- 1 teaspoon ground cinnamon

Instructions:

1. Preheat your oven to 200°F (95°C).

2. Arrange the apple slices in a single layer on a baking sheet lined with parchment paper.

3. Sprinkle the apple slices with ground cinnamon.

4. Bake for 2-3 hours, flipping halfway through, until the apple slices are crispy.

5. Let the apple chips cool completely before serving.

Nutritional Value:

80 calories | 0g fat | 0g saturated fat | 0mg cholesterol | 0mg sodium | 22g carbohydrate | 4g fiber | 16g sugar | 0g protein | 20mg calcium | 180mg potassium | 20mg phosphorus | 0.5mg iron | 0mcg vitamin D

Grilled Watermelon Triangles

Prep Time: 5 minutes | **Cooking Time:** 6 minutes | **Total Time:** 11 minutes | **Serving:** 4 | **Difficulty:** Easy

Ingredients:

- 1 small seedless watermelon, cut into 1-inch thick triangles

- 2 tablespoons honey or maple syrup (optional)

- Fresh mint leaves for garnish (optional)

Instructions:

1. Preheat your grill to medium-high heat.

2. If using, brush the watermelon triangles with honey or maple syrup.

3. Place the watermelon triangles on the grill and cook for 2-3 minutes on each side, until grill marks appear and the watermelon is slightly caramelized.

4. Serve warm, garnished with fresh mint leaves if desired.

Nutritional Value:

70 calories | 0g fat | 0g saturated fat | 0mg cholesterol | 0mg sodium | 18g carbohydrate | 1g fiber | 16g sugar | 1g protein | 10mg calcium | 170mg potassium | 20mg phosphorus | 0mg iron | 0mcg vitamin D

Baked Pear Halves

Prep Time: 10 minutes | **Cooking Time:** 25 minutes | **Total Time:** 35 minutes | **Serving:** 4 | **Difficulty:** Easy

Ingredients:

- 4 ripe pears, halved and cored
- 2 tablespoons honey or maple syrup
- 1 teaspoon ground cinnamon
- 1/4 teaspoon ground nutmeg (optional)

Instructions:

1. Preheat your oven to 375°F (190°C).

2. Place the pear halves cut side up in a baking dish.

3. Drizzle the pears with honey or maple syrup and sprinkle with ground cinnamon and nutmeg (if using).

4. Bake for 20-25 minutes, or until the pears are tender and caramelized.

5. Serve warm.

Nutritional Value:

150 calories | 0g fat | 0g saturated fat | 0mg cholesterol | 0mg sodium | 40g carbohydrate | 6g fiber | 28g sugar | 1g protein | 20mg calcium | 200mg potassium | 40mg phosphorus | 0.5mg iron | 0mcg vitamin D

Grilled Plum Halves

Prep Time: 5 minutes | **Cooking Time:** 6 minutes | **Total Time:** 11 minutes | **Serving:** 4 | **Difficulty:** Easy

Ingredients:

- 4 ripe plums, halved and pitted
- 2 tablespoons honey or maple syrup
- 1 teaspoon ground cinnamon

Instructions:

1. Preheat your grill to medium heat.

2. In a small bowl, mix together the honey or maple syrup and ground cinnamon.

3. Brush the cut sides of the plums with the honey mixture.

4. Place the plums cut side down on the grill and cook for 3-4 minutes, until grill marks appear and the plums are slightly softened.

5. Serve warm.

Nutritional Value:

80 calories | 0g fat | 0g saturated fat | 0mg cholesterol | 0mg sodium | 21g carbohydrate | 2g fiber | 18g sugar | 1g protein | 10mg calcium | 180mg potassium | 20mg phosphorus | 0.5mg iron | 0mcg vitamin D

Grilled Apricot Halves

Prep Time: 5 minutes | **Cooking Time:** 6 minutes | **Total Time:** 11 minutes | **Serving:** 4 | **Difficulty:** Easy

Ingredients:

- 4 ripe apricots, halved and pitted
- 2 tablespoons honey or maple syrup
- 1 teaspoon ground cinnamon

Instructions:

1. Preheat your grill to medium heat.

2. In a small bowl, mix together the honey or maple syrup and ground cinnamon.

3. Brush the cut sides of the apricots with the honey mixture.

4. Place the apricots cut side down on the grill and cook for 3-4 minutes, until grill marks appear and the apricots are slightly softened.

5. Serve warm.

Nutritional Value:

70 calories | 0g fat | 0g saturated fat | 0mg cholesterol | 0mg sodium | 18g carbohydrate | 2g fiber | 15g sugar | 1g protein | 10mg calcium | 180mg potassium | 20mg phosphorus | 0.5mg iron | 0mcg vitamin D

Grilled Cantaloupe Wedges

Prep Time: 5 minutes | **Cooking Time:** 6 minutes | **Total Time:** 11 minutes | **Serving:** 4 | **Difficulty:** Easy

Ingredients:

- 1 small cantaloupe, cut into wedges
- 2 tablespoons honey or maple syrup (optional)
- Fresh mint leaves for garnish (optional)

Instructions:

1. Preheat your grill to medium-high heat.

2. If using, brush the cantaloupe wedges with honey or maple syrup.

3. Place the cantaloupe wedges on the grill and cook for 2-3 minutes on each side, until grill marks appear and the cantaloupe is slightly caramelized.

4. Serve warm, garnished with fresh mint leaves if desired.

Nutritional Value:

60 calories | 0g fat | 0g saturated fat | 0mg cholesterol | 0mg sodium | 16g carbohydrate | 1g fiber | 14g sugar | 1g protein | 10mg calcium | 170mg potassium | 20mg phosphorus | 0mg iron | 0mcg vitamin D

Grilled Papaya Slices

Prep Time: 5 minutes | **Cooking Time:** 6 minutes | **Total Time:** 11 minutes | **Serving:** 4 | **Difficulty:** Easy

Ingredients:

- 1 ripe papaya, peeled, seeded, and cut into thick slices
- 2 tablespoons honey or maple syrup
- 1 teaspoon ground cinnamon

Instructions:

1. Preheat your grill to medium heat.

2. In a small bowl, mix together the honey or maple syrup and ground cinnamon.

3. Brush the papaya slices with the honey mixture.

4. Place the papaya slices on the grill and cook for 2-3 minutes on each side, until grill marks appear and the papaya is slightly caramelized.

5. Serve warm.

Nutritional Value:

100 calories | 0g fat | 0g saturated fat | 0mg cholesterol | 5mg sodium | 26g carbohydrate | 3g fiber | 18g sugar | 1g protein | 20mg calcium | 200mg potassium | 30mg phosphorus | 0.5mg iron | 0mcg vitamin D

Grilled Mango Cheeks

Prep Time: 5 minutes | **Cooking Time:** 6 minutes | **Total Time:** 11 minutes | **Serving:** 4 | **Difficulty:** Easy

Ingredients:

- 2 ripe mangoes, cheeks sliced off
- 2 tablespoons honey or maple syrup
- 1 teaspoon ground cinnamon

Instructions:

1. Preheat your grill to medium heat.

2. In a small bowl, mix together the honey or maple syrup and ground cinnamon.

3. Brush the mango cheeks with the honey mixture.

4. Place the mango cheeks on the grill and cook for 2-3 minutes on each side, until grill marks appear and the mango is slightly caramelized.

5. Serve warm.

Nutritional Value:

110 calories | 0g fat | 0g saturated fat | 0mg cholesterol | 5mg sodium | 28g carbohydrate | 3g fiber | 22g sugar | 1g protein | 20mg calcium | 200mg potassium | 30mg phosphorus | 0.5mg iron | 0mcg vitamin D

Grilled Honeydew Melon Wedges

Prep Time: 5 minutes | **Cooking Time:** 6 minutes | **Total Time:** 11 minutes | **Serving:** 4 | **Difficulty:** Easy

Ingredients:

- 1 small honeydew melon, cut into wedges
- 2 tablespoons honey or maple syrup (optional)
- Fresh mint leaves for garnish (optional)

Instructions:

1. Preheat your grill to medium-high heat.

2. If using, brush the honeydew melon wedges with honey or maple syrup.

3. Place the melon wedges on the grill and cook for 2-3 minutes on each side, until grill marks appear and the melon is slightly caramelized.

4. Serve warm, garnished with fresh mint leaves if desired.

Nutritional Value:

60 calories | 0g fat | 0g saturated fat | 0mg cholesterol | 0mg sodium | 15g carbohydrate | 1g fiber | 14g sugar | 1g protein | 10mg calcium | 160mg potassium | 20mg phosphorus | 0mg iron | 0mcg vitamin D

Grilled Starfruit Slices

Prep Time: 5 minutes | **Cooking Time:** 6 minutes | **Total Time:** 11 minutes | **Serving:** 4 | **Difficulty:** Easy

Ingredients:

- 2 ripe starfruits, sliced crosswise into 1/4-inch thick slices
- 2 tablespoons honey or maple syrup (optional)
- 1 teaspoon ground cinnamon (optional)

Instructions:

1. Preheat your grill to medium heat.

2. If using, brush the starfruit slices with honey or maple syrup and sprinkle with ground cinnamon.

3. Place the starfruit slices on the grill and cook for 2-3 minutes on each side, until grill marks appear and the starfruit is slightly caramelized.

4. Serve warm.

Nutritional Value:

50 calories | 0g fat | 0g saturated fat | 0mg cholesterol | 0mg sodium | 13g carbohydrate | 3g fiber | 8g sugar | 1g protein | 10mg calcium | 120mg potassium | 20mg phosphorus | 0mg iron | 0mcg vitamin D

Grilled Guava Halves

Prep Time: 5 minutes | **Cooking Time:** 6 minutes | **Total Time:** 11 minutes | **Serving:** 4 | **Difficulty:** Easy

Ingredients:

- 4 ripe guavas, halved and seeds removed
- 2 tablespoons honey or maple syrup
- 1 teaspoon ground cinnamon

Instructions:

1. Preheat your grill to medium heat.

2. In a small bowl, mix together the honey or maple syrup and ground cinnamon.

3. Brush the cut sides of the guava halves with the honey mixture.

4. Place the guava halves cut side down on the grill and cook for 3-4 minutes, until grill marks appear and the guava is slightly softened.

5. Serve warm.

Nutritional Value:

80 calories | 0g fat | 0g saturated fat | 0mg cholesterol | 0mg sodium | 20g carbohydrate | 3g fiber | 15g sugar | 1g protein | 20mg calcium | 150mg potassium | 30mg phosphorus | 0.5mg iron | 0mcg vitamin D

Grilled Dragon Fruit Slices

Prep Time: 5 minutes | **Cooking Time:** 6 minutes | **Total Time:** 11 minutes | **Serving:** 4 | **Difficulty:** Easy

Ingredients:

- 2 ripe dragon fruits, peeled and sliced into rounds
- 2 tablespoons honey or maple syrup
- 1 teaspoon ground cinnamon (optional)

Instructions:

1. Preheat your grill to medium heat.

2. If using, brush the dragon fruit slices with honey or maple syrup and sprinkle with ground cinnamon.

3. Place the dragon fruit slices on the grill and cook for 2-3 minutes on each side, until grill marks appear and the fruit is slightly caramelized.

4. Serve warm.

Nutritional Value:

90 calories | 0g fat | 0g saturated fat | 0mg cholesterol | 0mg sodium | 23g carbohydrate | 3g fiber | 17g sugar | 2g protein | 10mg calcium | 200mg potassium | 30mg phosphorus | 0.5mg iron | 0mcg vitamin D

Grilled Kiwi Halves

Prep Time: 5 minutes | **Cooking Time:** 6 minutes | **Total Time:** 11 minutes | **Serving:** 4 | **Difficulty:** Easy

Ingredients:

- 4 ripe kiwis, halved and peeled

- 2 tablespoons honey or maple syrup (optional)

- 1 teaspoon ground cinnamon (optional)

Instructions:

1. Preheat your grill to medium heat.

2. If using, brush the cut sides of the kiwi halves with honey or maple syrup and sprinkle with ground cinnamon.

3. Place the kiwi halves cut side down on the grill and cook for 2-3 minutes,

until grill marks appear and the kiwi is slightly softened.

4. Serve warm.

Nutritional Value:

70 calories | 0g fat | 0g saturated fat | 0mg cholesterol | 0mg sodium | 18g carbohydrate | 3g fiber | 12g sugar | 1g protein | 20mg calcium | 180mg potassium | 20mg phosphorus | 0.5mg iron | 0mcg vitamin D

Grilled Lychee Halves

Prep Time: 5 minutes | **Cooking Time:** 6 minutes | **Total Time:** 11 minutes | **Serving:** 4 | **Difficulty:** Easy

Ingredients:

- 20 ripe lychees, peeled, pitted, and halved

- 2 tablespoons honey or maple syrup (optional)

- 1 teaspoon ground cinnamon (optional)

Instructions:

1. Preheat your grill to medium heat.

2. If using, brush the lychee halves with honey or maple syrup and sprinkle with ground cinnamon.

3. Place the lychee halves on the grill and cook for 2-3 minutes, until grill marks appear and the lychee is slightly caramelized.

4. Serve warm.

Nutritional Value:

60 calories | 0g fat | 0g saturated fat | 0mg cholesterol | 0mg sodium | 16g carbohydrate | 2g fiber | 12g sugar | 1g protein | 10mg calcium | 120mg potassium | 20mg phosphorus | 0mg iron | 0mcg vitamin D

Grilled Persimmon Wedges

Prep Time: 5 minutes | **Cooking Time:** 6 minutes | **Total Time:** 11 minutes | **Serving:** 4 | **Difficulty:** Easy

Ingredients:

- 2 ripe persimmons, sliced into wedges
- 2 tablespoons honey or maple syrup (optional)
- 1 teaspoon ground cinnamon

Instructions:

1. Preheat your grill to medium heat.

2. If using, brush the persimmon wedges with honey or maple syrup and sprinkle with ground cinnamon.

3. Place the persimmon wedges on the grill and cook for 2-3 minutes on each side, until grill marks appear and the persimmons are slightly softened.

4. Serve warm.

Nutritional Value:

70 calories | 0g fat | 0g saturated fat | 0mg cholesterol | 0mg sodium | 18g carbohydrate | 3g fiber | 15g sugar | 1g protein | 20mg calcium | 200mg potassium | 30mg phosphorus | 0.5mg iron | 0mcg vitamin D

Snacks and Light Bites

Baked Eggplant Slices

Prep Time: 10 minutes | **Cooking Time:** 25 minutes | **Total Time:** 35 minutes | **Serving:** 4 | **Difficulty:** Easy

Ingredients:

- 1 large eggplant, sliced into 1/2-inch rounds
- 2 tablespoons olive oil
- 1 teaspoon garlic powder
- 1 teaspoon dried oregano
- Salt and pepper, to taste

Instructions:

1. Preheat your oven to 400°F (200°C).
2. In a large bowl, toss the eggplant slices with olive oil, garlic powder, oregano, salt, and pepper.
3. Arrange the slices in a single layer on a baking sheet lined with parchment paper.
4. Bake for 20-25 minutes, flipping halfway through, until the eggplant slices are golden brown and tender.
5. Serve hot.

Nutritional Value:
100 calories | 7g fat | 1g saturated fat | 0mg cholesterol | 160mg sodium | 9g carbohydrate | 4g fiber | 4g sugar | 2g protein | 20mg calcium | 250mg potassium | 50mg phosphorus | 0.5mg iron | 0mcg vitamin D

Baked Acorn Squash

Prep Time: 10 minutes | **Cooking Time:** 35 minutes | **Total Time:** 45 minutes | **Serving:** 4 | **Difficulty:** Easy

Ingredients:

- 1 medium acorn squash, halved and seeds removed
- 2 tablespoons olive oil
- 1 teaspoon ground cinnamon
- 1 tablespoon maple syrup (optional)
- Salt and pepper, to taste

Instructions:

1. Preheat your oven to 400°F (200°C).
2. Cut the acorn squash into wedges or leave in halves, depending on preference.
3. In a small bowl, mix together olive oil, cinnamon, maple syrup (if using), salt, and pepper.
4. Brush the mixture over the squash wedges or halves.

5. Place the squash on a baking sheet lined with parchment paper, cut side down.

6. Bake for 30-35 minutes, or until the squash is tender when pierced with a fork.

7. Serve hot.

Nutritional Value:
130 calories | 7g fat | 1g saturated fat | 0mg cholesterol | 20mg sodium | 17g carbohydrate | 3g fiber | 5g sugar | 1g protein | 40mg calcium | 400mg potassium | 40mg phosphorus | 0.5mg iron | 0mcg vitamin D

Baked Zucchini Boats

Prep Time: 10 minutes | **Cooking Time:** 20 minutes | **Total Time:** 30 minutes | **Serving:** 4 | **Difficulty:** Easy

Ingredients:

- 4 medium zucchinis, halved lengthwise and seeds scooped out
- 2 tablespoons olive oil
- 1 garlic clove, minced
- 1/4 cup grated Parmesan cheese (optional)
- 1 teaspoon dried basil
- Salt and pepper, to taste

Instructions:

1. Preheat your oven to 375°F (190°C).

2. In a small bowl, mix together the olive oil, minced garlic, dried basil, salt, and pepper.

3. Brush the mixture onto the zucchini halves.

4. If using, sprinkle the grated Parmesan cheese over the zucchini.

5. Place the zucchini boats on a baking sheet lined with parchment paper.

6. Bake for 18-20 minutes, or until the zucchini is tender.

7. Serve hot.

Nutritional Value:
100 calories | 7g fat | 1g saturated fat | 0mg cholesterol | 160mg sodium | 7g carbohydrate | 2g fiber | 4g sugar | 2g protein | 30mg calcium | 350mg potassium | 40mg phosphorus | 0.5mg iron | 0mcg vitamin D

Baked Parsnip Chips

Prep Time: 10 minutes | **Cooking Time:** 20 minutes | **Total Time:** 30 minutes | **Serving:** 4 | **Difficulty:** Easy

Ingredients:

- 4 large parsnips, peeled and thinly sliced
- 2 tablespoons olive oil
- 1 teaspoon garlic powder
- 1 teaspoon smoked paprika

- Salt and pepper, to taste

Instructions:

1. Preheat your oven to 375°F (190°C).

2. In a large bowl, toss the parsnip slices with olive oil, garlic powder, smoked paprika, salt, and pepper.

3. Spread the slices in a single layer on a baking sheet lined with parchment paper.

4. Bake for 15-20 minutes, flipping halfway through, until the chips are crispy and golden brown.

5. Serve hot.

Nutritional Value:

120 calories | 7g fat | 1g saturated fat | 0mg cholesterol | 160mg sodium | 14g carbohydrate | 4g fiber | 4g sugar | 1g protein | 30mg calcium | 300mg potassium | 50mg phosphorus | 0.5mg iron | 0mcg vitamin D

Baked Plantain Slices

Prep Time: 5 minutes | **Cooking Time:** 25 minutes | **Total Time:** 30 minutes | **Serving:** 4 | **Difficulty:** Easy

Ingredients:

- 2 large ripe plantains, peeled and sliced into 1/2-inch rounds

- 2 tablespoons olive oil

- Salt, to taste

- Ground cinnamon (optional)

Instructions:

1. Preheat your oven to 400°F (200°C).

2. In a large bowl, toss the plantain slices with olive oil and salt. If desired, add a sprinkle of ground cinnamon.

3. Arrange the plantain slices in a single layer on a baking sheet lined with parchment paper.

4. Bake for 20-25 minutes, flipping halfway through, until the plantains are golden brown and crispy.

5. Serve hot.

Nutritional Value:

180 calories | 7g fat | 1g saturated fat | 0mg cholesterol | 160mg sodium | 31g carbohydrate | 2g fiber | 14g sugar | 1g protein | 10mg calcium | 350mg potassium | 30mg phosphorus | 0.5mg iron | 0mcg vitamin D

Managing Flare-Ups with Food

Common Foods to Avoid During Flare-Ups

1. **Spicy Foods**

   - Hot peppers (chili, jalapeño)

   - Hot sauces

   - Spicy seasonings (cayenne, paprika)

2. **Acidic Foods**

   - Citrus fruits (oranges, lemons, limes, grapefruits)

   - Tomato products (tomato sauce, ketchup, salsa)

   - Vinegar-based foods (pickles, salad dressings)

3. **Caffeinated Beverages**

   - Coffee (regular and decaffeinated)

   - Black tea

   - Energy drinks

   - Cola and other caffeinated sodas

4. **Carbonated Beverages**

   - Sodas

   - Sparkling water

   - Carbonated energy drinks

5. **Alcoholic Beverages**

   - Beer

   - Wine

   - Liquor (whiskey, vodka, rum)

6. **Fried and Greasy Foods**

   - French fries

   - Fried chicken

   - Doughnuts

   - Potato chips

7. **Dairy Products (for those who are lactose intolerant)**

   - Whole milk

   - Cream

   - Full-fat cheese

   - Ice cream

8. **Chocolate and Sweets**

   - Chocolate bars

   - Chocolate-flavored drinks

   - Pastries and cakes with chocolate

9. **Processed and Red Meats**

   - Bacon

   - Sausages

   - Salami

   - Hot dogs

10. **High-Fat Foods**

   - Butter

   - Creamy sauces

   - High-fat cuts of meat (ribeye, pork belly)

11. **High-Salt Foods**

   - Salted snacks (pretzels, chips)

- Processed meats

- Canned soups and broths with high sodium content

12. **Artificial Sweeteners**

- Aspartame

- Saccharin

- Sucralose

13. **Nuts and Seeds (especially if they are hard to digest)**

- Almonds

- Walnuts

- Sunflower seeds

- Sesame seeds

14. **Legumes (for some individuals)**

- Beans (kidney, black, pinto)

- Lentils

- Chickpeas

15. **Raw Vegetables (can be hard to digest for some)**

- Broccoli

- Cauliflower

- Bell peppers

- Onions

16. **Certain Fruits**

- Berries (strawberries, raspberries)

- Pineapple

- Grapes

17. **Garlic and Onions (especially raw)**

- Raw garlic

- Raw onions

- Garlic powder

18. **Mint and Peppermint Products**

- Mint-flavored candies

- Peppermint tea

- Mint-flavored gum

19. **Gluten-Containing Foods (for those with gluten sensitivity)**

- Bread

- Pasta

- Cereals

- Baked goods

20. **Artificial Preservatives and Additives**

- MSG (monosodium glutamate)

- Nitrates/nitrites

- Sulfites

Keeping a Food Diary for Symptom Management

Maintaining a food diary can be an invaluable tool for managing ulcer symptoms. By tracking what you eat and how you feel afterward, you can identify foods that may trigger flare-ups and adjust your diet accordingly. Here's how to effectively keep a food diary:

1. Choose Your Method

- **Notebook:** A simple notebook is easy to carry and allows you to jot down meals, symptoms, and any relevant notes.

- **Mobile Apps:** There are various apps available that can help you track your food intake, symptoms, and even nutrient content. Examples include MyFitnessPal or a simple notes app.

- **Spreadsheet:** A digital spreadsheet can help you organize your entries in a structured format, allowing for easier analysis.

2. What to Record

- **Date and Time:** Note the date and time of each meal, snack, or drink.

- **Detailed Food Intake:** Write down everything you consume, including meals, snacks, beverages, and even small bites or sips. Be specific about portion sizes, ingredients, and preparation methods.

- **Symptoms:** Record any symptoms you experience after eating, including their severity and timing. Common symptoms to track include:

  - Stomach pain

  - Heartburn

  - Nausea

  - Bloating

  - Indigestion

- **Other Factors:** Include any other factors that might affect your symptoms, such as stress levels, sleep quality, physical activity, and medications taken.

3. Analyzing Your Entries

- **Identify Patterns:** After a few weeks, review your diary to identify any patterns between certain foods or drinks and the onset of symptoms.

- **Food Triggers:** Look for specific foods that consistently cause symptoms and consider eliminating or reducing them in your diet.

- **Time of Day:** Note if symptoms are worse at certain times of the day or after specific meals, which might suggest when your stomach is more sensitive.

- **Portion Sizes:** Consider whether the quantity of food impacts your symptoms. Sometimes smaller, more frequent meals may be easier on the stomach.

4. Adjusting Your Diet

- **Eliminate Triggers:** Based on your findings, gradually eliminate foods that seem to trigger symptoms. Be mindful to do this one food at a time to accurately identify the culprits.

- **Introduce New Foods Slowly:** When trying new foods, introduce them one at a time and record how they affect you.

- **Monitor Changes:** Continue to track your symptoms as you make dietary changes, noting improvements or any new triggers that emerge.

5. Share with Your Healthcare Provider

- **Consultation:** Share your food diary with your healthcare provider or dietitian. They can offer insights and suggest further dietary adjustments based on your symptoms and the diary.

- **Adjust Treatment:** Your healthcare provider may adjust your treatment plan based on the patterns and triggers identified in your diary.

6. Long-Term Use

- **Ongoing Management:** Continue using the food diary as long as needed to manage your symptoms. It's particularly useful during periods of flare-ups or when trying new treatments or diets.

- **Periodic Review:** Even after your symptoms improve, consider reviewing your food diary periodically to ensure you're maintaining a symptom-free diet.

Frequently Asked Questions

1. What foods should I avoid if I have an ulcer?

Avoid foods that can increase stomach acid production or irritate the stomach lining. Common culprits include:

- Spicy foods (e.g., chili, hot sauce)
- Acidic foods (e.g., citrus fruits, tomatoes, vinegar)
- Caffeinated beverages (e.g., coffee, tea, soda)
- Alcohol
- Fried and greasy foods
- Chocolate
- High-fat dairy products

2. Can certain foods help heal my ulcer?

While no single food can heal an ulcer, some foods may support healing by reducing irritation and providing essential nutrients. These include:

- Foods high in fiber, such as oats, barley, and beans, which may help reduce stomach acid production.
- Lean proteins like chicken, turkey, and fish.
- Non-acidic fruits like bananas and melons.
- Vegetables like carrots, sweet potatoes, and squash.

3. Is it okay to drink milk if I have an ulcer?

Milk was once thought to soothe ulcers by coating the stomach lining. However, it can actually stimulate the production of stomach acid, which may worsen symptoms. It's best to consume milk in moderation or choose low-fat or lactose-free options if tolerated.

4. Should I avoid all acidic foods if I have an ulcer?

Not all acidic foods will necessarily trigger symptoms for everyone with an ulcer. It's important to identify your own triggers by keeping a food diary. However, it's generally advisable to limit foods like citrus fruits, tomatoes, and vinegar during flare-ups.

5. Can stress really affect my ulcer, and how should I adjust my diet accordingly?

Stress can increase stomach acid production and exacerbate ulcer symptoms. During stressful periods, stick to a bland, low-acid diet, and incorporate stress-reduction techniques such as mindful eating, which encourages slower eating and better digestion.

6. Is it necessary to eat bland food if I have an ulcer?

During flare-ups, bland foods can help minimize irritation to the stomach lining. Focus on easily digestible foods like bananas, oatmeal, plain rice, steamed vegetables, and lean proteins. Once symptoms improve, you can gradually reintroduce more variety into your diet.

7. How can I manage my symptoms when eating out?

When dining out, choose restaurants that offer simple, grilled, or steamed dishes. Avoid spicy, fried, or heavily seasoned foods. Ask for sauces and dressings on the side, and opt for smaller portions to avoid overeating.

8. Can I drink coffee or tea if I have an ulcer?

Caffeinated beverages like coffee and black tea can increase stomach acid production and irritate the stomach lining. It's best to avoid them or switch to herbal teas like chamomile or ginger, which may soothe the stomach.

9. How often should I eat if I have an ulcer?

Eating smaller, more frequent meals (5-6 times a day) can help keep stomach acid levels stable and prevent irritation. Avoid large meals, especially close to bedtime, to reduce the risk of nighttime symptoms.

10. What should I do if certain foods seem to make my symptoms worse?

If you notice that certain foods consistently trigger symptoms, it's best to avoid them. Keeping a food diary can help you track your diet and identify specific foods that cause discomfort. Gradually eliminate these foods from your diet and consult with a healthcare provider or dietitian for personalized advice.

11. Can I still eat fruits and vegetables with an ulcer?

Yes, fruits and vegetables are important for overall health. Choose low-acid options like bananas, melons, cooked carrots, and spinach. Avoid raw vegetables during flare-ups, as they can be harder to digest.

12. Are there any supplements I should take or avoid with an ulcer?

Consult with your healthcare provider before taking any supplements. While some supplements like probiotics may help with gut health, others, such as NSAIDs (non-steroidal anti-inflammatory drugs), should be avoided as they can worsen ulcers.

13. How long should I stick to a specific diet after my ulcer symptoms improve?

Even after symptoms improve, it's important to maintain a balanced diet to prevent future flare-ups. Gradually reintroduce foods and monitor your symptoms. A long-term focus on a healthy, ulcer-friendly diet can support overall digestive health.

14. Can alcohol worsen ulcer symptoms?

Yes, alcohol can irritate the stomach lining and increase acid production, potentially worsening ulcer symptoms. It's advisable to avoid alcohol or limit intake significantly.

15. What are some safe snacks I can eat if I have an ulcer?

Safe snack options include:

- Plain crackers
- Yogurt (if tolerated)
- Applesauce
- Rice cakes
- Smoothies made with non-acidic fruits and yogurt

16. Is it okay to eat spicy foods if my symptoms are under control?

Spicy foods can irritate the stomach lining, so it's best to avoid them even if your symptoms are under control. However, you may experiment with mild spices like ginger or turmeric in small amounts to see how your body reacts.

Myths and Misconceptions

1. Myth: Spicy Foods Cause Ulcers

- **Fact:** While spicy foods can irritate the stomach lining and worsen ulcer symptoms, they do not cause ulcers. The primary causes of ulcers are infections with *Helicobacter pylori* (H. pylori) bacteria and the prolonged use of non-steroidal anti-inflammatory drugs (NSAIDs) like ibuprofen and aspirin.

2. Myth: Milk Heals Ulcers

- **Fact:** Milk was once believed to soothe ulcers because it can temporarily neutralize stomach acid. However, milk also stimulates the production of stomach acid, which can exacerbate ulcer symptoms. It's best to consume milk in moderation or opt for low-fat options if tolerated.

3. Myth: Stress Alone Causes Ulcers

- **Fact:** Stress does not directly cause ulcers, but it can exacerbate symptoms and delay healing. The most common causes of ulcers are *H. pylori* infection and NSAID use. However, managing stress is still important for overall health and can help reduce the impact of ulcer symptoms.

4. Myth: Only Certain People Get Ulcers

- **Fact:** Anyone can develop an ulcer, regardless of age, gender, or lifestyle. However, certain factors increase the risk, such as *H. pylori* infection, frequent use of NSAIDs, smoking, and excessive alcohol consumption.

5. Myth: You Should Avoid All Acidic Foods if You Have an Ulcer

- **Fact:** Not all acidic foods need to be avoided. Some acidic foods, like citrus fruits, can irritate the stomach lining and worsen symptoms for some people, but others may tolerate them well. It's important to identify your own triggers and avoid only those specific foods that cause discomfort.

6. Myth: Ulcers Are a Result of Poor Diet

- **Fact:** While diet can influence the severity of ulcer symptoms, ulcers are not directly caused by poor diet. *H. pylori* infection and NSAID use are the primary causes. However, a balanced diet can help manage symptoms and promote healing.

7. Myth: You Should Eat Bland Food All the Time If You Have an Ulcer

- **Fact:** Bland foods can be helpful during flare-ups, but you don't have to stick to a bland diet permanently. Once symptoms are under control, you can gradually reintroduce a variety of foods while monitoring how your body responds.

8. Myth: Ulcers Are Always Painful

- **Fact:** While pain is a common symptom of ulcers, not everyone experiences pain. Some people may have ulcers and not show any symptoms, which is why it's important to seek medical advice if you have risk factors or notice any changes in your digestive health.

9. Myth: Drinking Alcohol Can Help Numb Ulcer Pain

- **Fact:** Alcohol can actually worsen ulcer symptoms by irritating the stomach lining and increasing acid production. It's best to avoid alcohol if you have an ulcer.

10. Myth: Only Adults Get Ulcers

- **Fact:** Ulcers can affect people of all ages, including children. While less common in children, ulcers can occur due to *H. pylori* infection or the use of certain medications.

11. Myth: All Antacids Cure Ulcers

- **Fact:** Antacids can provide temporary relief from ulcer symptoms by neutralizing stomach acid, but they do not cure ulcers. Proper treatment usually involves antibiotics (for *H. pylori* infection), proton pump inhibitors (PPIs), or other medications prescribed by a healthcare provider.

12. Myth: Once You Have an Ulcer, You Will Always Have It

- **Fact:** With proper treatment, most ulcers can heal completely. However, it's important to follow your healthcare provider's recommendations and make necessary lifestyle changes to prevent recurrence.

13. Myth: You Can't Eat Fiber If You Have an Ulcer

- **Fact:** While high-fiber foods may be harder to digest during a flare-up, fiber is generally beneficial for digestive health. Soluble fiber, in particular, can be soothing for the digestive tract. Gradually reintroduce fiber-rich foods like oats, barley, and cooked vegetables as your symptoms improve.

14. Myth: If You're Not in Pain, Your Ulcer is Healed

- **Fact:** Absence of pain doesn't necessarily mean an ulcer has healed. Some ulcers may be asymptomatic or have fluctuating symptoms. It's important to follow through with treatment and have follow-up evaluations to ensure healing.

15. Myth: You Can Diagnose an Ulcer Based on Symptoms Alone

- **Fact:** Symptoms of an ulcer can be similar to those of other digestive conditions, so it's essential to get a proper diagnosis from a healthcare provider. Diagnostic tests such as endoscopy or testing for *H. pylori* are often necessary to confirm the presence of an ulcer.

Conclusion

Embarking on the journey to manage your ulcer and maintain a healthy lifestyle is a significant step toward better well-being. It's a path that requires dedication, awareness, and a commitment to making informed choices about your diet and overall health.

Encouragement for Continuing Your Health Journey

Living with an ulcer can be challenging, but it's important to remember that with the right strategies, you can lead a comfortable and fulfilling life. Every meal choice, every stress management technique, and every healthy habit you adopt brings you closer to achieving better digestive health.

- **Stay Informed:** Knowledge is your strongest ally. Continue to learn about your condition, listen to your body, and stay updated on the latest advice from healthcare professionals.

- **Be Patient:** Healing and symptom management take time. Progress might be slow, but every small step counts. Celebrate your successes, no matter how small they may seem.

- **Seek Support:** You are not alone in this journey. Whether it's friends, family, or a support group, surround yourself with people who understand and support your health goals.

- **Keep a Positive Mindset:** Focus on the improvements you make rather than the setbacks. A positive outlook can greatly influence your overall well-being and help you stay motivated.

Final Thoughts on Maintaining an Ulcer-Friendly Lifestyle

Maintaining an ulcer-friendly lifestyle is about more than just managing symptoms—it's about creating a balanced, nourishing, and sustainable way of living that supports your long-term health.

- **Prioritize Balance:** An ulcer-friendly diet doesn't mean deprivation. Enjoy a variety of foods that are gentle on your stomach and provide the nutrients you need to thrive.

- **Make Mindful Choices:** Pay attention to how different foods and habits affect your body. Use this awareness to make choices that promote healing and comfort.

- **Adapt and Adjust:** Your body's needs may change over time. Be flexible in adapting your diet and lifestyle to meet those needs, especially during periods of stress or flare-ups.

- **Integrate Wellness:** Beyond diet, consider how other aspects of your life—such as stress management, sleep, and physical activity—contribute to your overall health. A holistic approach can provide greater benefits.

As you continue your health journey, remember that the choices you make today lay the foundation for a healthier future. Stay committed to your well-being, and know that with each day, you're building a lifestyle that supports not just your ulcer management but your overall quality of life.

Conversion Table

Measurement	U.S. (Standard/Imperial)	Metric	Notes
Volume			
1 teaspoon	1 tsp	5 ml	
1 tablespoon	1 tbsp	15 ml	3 teaspoons
1/4 cup	4 tbsp	60 ml	
1/3 cup	5 tbsp + 1 tsp	80 ml	
1/2 cup	8 tbsp	120 ml	
2/3 cup	10 tbsp + 2 tsp	160 ml	
3/4 cup	12 tbsp	180 ml	
1 cup	16 tbsp	240 ml	
1 pint	2 cups	480 ml	
1 quart	4 cups	960 ml	
1 gallon	16 cups	3.8 liters	4 quarts

Weight			
1 ounce	1 oz	28 g	
4 ounces	4 oz	113 g	1/4 pound
8 ounces	8 oz	227 g	1/2 pound
12 ounces	12 oz	340 g	3/4 pound
16 ounces	16 oz	454 g	1 pound

Length

1/4 inch	1/4 in	0.6 cm	
1/2 inch	1/2 in	1.3 cm	
3/4 inch	3/4 in	1.9 cm	
1 inch	1 in	2.5 cm	
2 inches	2 in	5 cm	
4 inches	4 in	10 cm	

Temperature

250°F	250°F	120°C	Low heat
300°F	300°F	150°C	Moderate heat
350°F	350°F	180°C	Moderate heat
375°F	375°F	190°C	Moderate-high heat
400°F	400°F	200°C	High heat
425°F	425°F	220°C	High heat
450°F	450°F	230°C	Very high heat

Made in the USA
Thornton, CO
02/17/25 15:28:17

25b9d9ae-1ffb-42c2-86ca-dded7a7e5281R02